POSTURE

Everything You Need to Improve Posture in Just a Few Minutes Per Day

(The Complete Guide to Safe and Effective Exercises for Osteoporosis and Posture)

Dennis Powers

Published By Dennis Powers

Dennis Powers

Posture: Everything You Need to Improve Posture in Just a Few Minutes Per Day (The Complete Guide to Safe and Effective Exercises for Osteoporosis and Posture)

ISBN 978-1-77485-399-3

Legal & Disclaimer

The information contained in this book is not designed to replace or take the place of any form of medicine or professional medical advice. The information in this book has been provided for educational and entertainment purposes only.

The information contained in this book has been compiled from sources deemed reliable, and it is accurate to the best of the Author's knowledge; however, the Author cannot guarantee its accuracy and validity and cannot be held liable for any errors or omissions. Changes are periodically made to this book. You must consult your doctor or get professional medical advice before using any of the suggested remedies, techniques, or information in this book.

TABLE OF CONTENTS

Introduction

Have you ever thought about the numerous different positions we put our bodies in during the day? If you're standing, sitting in a jog, walking, or a walk bent over to grab something as well as standing up with your arms stretched out when replacing a lightbulb your body can be bent, tied to, and twisting in various postures. Luckily, every one of us has the strength to handle all of the everyday stresses however, sometimes our bodies are stretched to the edge, leading to injuries. Three main reasons for injury:

1. Repetitive movement

2. Traumatic movement

3. Insufficiency of positioning for long periods

We are affixed to the daily demands that require us to do the same repetitive movements perform body mechanics in a way which cause strains and pains and force us into dangerous, unnatural positions, it is essential to become aware of the causes and take action accordingly. Understanding how an injury develops by contemplating the postures we are in, we will have the ability to avoid discomfort by altering our routines.

Chapter 1: The Truth About Back Pain

It doesn't matter if it's severe or not when back pain strikes you, your everyday routines will definitely be affected. In reality, as per studies, back pains are one of the most common reasons that employees are unable to job, and it's next to respiratory ailments as the most common reason patients visit their doctor.

A. What could be the cause of back discomfort?

According to specialists, back pains tend to be the result of injuries, sprains, or an irritation of a nerve. But, it is important to keep in mind that back pains can be an indication of an even more serious health issue.

Here are a few reasons for back discomfort:

Back Strain: Lifting weighty objects may cause muscles of your back to relax or tear, causing lower back discomfort.

Patients who are suffering from back strain may experience pain, muscle spasms, or even a painful ache according to the severity and severity of injury.

Intervertebral Degenerative Disc Disease- back pain is among the signs of this disc injury which may affect people who are younger than 20 years of age. The discs between vertebrae in the lower back become damaged that in turn causes pain and irritation to the lower back and sciatica that causes discomfort from the hips down to the lower legs.

Arthritis- sufferers from arthritis (either osteoarthritis or rheumatoidarthritis) can be prone to suffering lower back pains.

Muscle Irritation- people who take part in sports or other strenuous activitiesoften suffer from lower back pain caused by muscular irritation or myofascial discomfort. Incorrect posture and injuries caused by an auto accident can also be cited as the reason for lower back pain.

In recent years experts have noticed an increase in back pain-related complaints because of stress. When you are stressed, your muscles in the back get tight, causing painful spasms in the back.

B. What are the different kinds of back discomfort?

Back pain is typically classified in two kinds of pain, which are acute as well as chronic. Back pains are classified as acute when the pain is directly linked in any way to muscle injury or damage or when the pain lasts for less than 3 months. The pain that is caused by degenerative disc diseases is classified as chronic or if there is a persistent pain that persists until treatment.

C. Who is susceptible to back pain?

Many people have, at some time in their lives, been affected by back discomfort. But there are some risk factors that make people more prone to back pain. These are:

1. If you are overweight or obese- carrying extra body weight may cause tension on the spine which could cause back pain.

2. Women who are pregnant- again, the additional burden of carrying a newborn could cause women to suffer intense back discomforts.

3.Smokers, in addition to being susceptible to chronic respiratory ailments, smoking cigarettes may also result in back tissue damage and osteoporosis.

4.People who always feel stressed- the discomfort you feel in your back when the office become chaotic is due to the muscles tightening when you're stressed.

5.People who are taking medicationsThere are some drugs that are corticosteroids that could cause the bones to weaken particularly when taken over longer periods of time.

D. What is back pain identified?

As I said earlier, most people suffer from back pain. You can ignore the discomfort or apply ice in particular if you believe that the discomfort is result of poor posture for a prolonged duration, improper posture of moving heavy things, or. If the pain continues or is getting worse even though you've tried all sorts of treatments, then I suggest you immediately consult your doctor.

It's crucial to inform your physician know about the discomfort you're experiencing in order to rule out any more grave health issues.

If you see your physician, you'll be asked a variety of questions, such as "How long have you been experiencing discomfort?", "Do you experience pain when lying, sitting or standing?", or "How do you feel the pain?", etc.

It is also possible to go through a series of tests like an x-ray MRI and myelogram, so your doctor can provide the proper diagnosis and treatment for back discomfort.

Chapter 2: Around The Neck

"The body is in a state of relaxation to nature"

Prewords

Neck pain is a category of conditions that are most prevalent. The most common are people who work in front of their computer. A lot of people feel neck pain which extends to the shoulders, or maybe down to an upper arm. Some suffer from a sharper pain in the base of the skull that can cause migraines and headaches.

Tension caused by the static posture of the neck and arms frequently encountered in bus drivers, office workers and similar tasks can also cause injuries and ailments, including radiating discomfort in your arm (thoracic outlet syndrome TOS) and tension migraine, headache degenerative changes, or disc herniation. All of these conditions will be addressed in this book, in their own chapters.

If you're reading about your neck, I would like you to keep in mind that shoulder and neck muscles function a lot in tandem and connect to one another. A large portion of neck examination and rehabilitation also involves the shoulders ' function. This is why I urge readers to check out my previous publication "Free of shoulder discomfort" in order to gain the full picture of how the shoulder and neck pains. This will help you know how everything is connected and the rehabilitation process becomes better and more efficient.

Basic understanding of anatomy

As is the norm, we begin with anatomical anatomy and the structure of neck. This will give an understanding of the rehabilitation process for different injuries.

The spinal column

The cervical spine is comprised of seven vertebrae. The vertebrae that are at the top of the spine that the head is resting is known as the Atlas vertebrae, while the 7th is known as Prominens due to the fact that it is the vertebra with the highest protrusion throughout the entire spinal column. Necks are further split into two groups: the neck's upper and lower joints. They are separated in this manner due to their distinct functions, as they execute certain actions.

The neck's upper joint actually only one joint that connects your head as well as the vertebra first, Atlas. The majority of flexing movements are performed forwards and backwards along with lesser mobility during the side bends and rotations.

Lower neck joints lies situated between Atlas along with the vertebrae that is second, Axis. This is, in contrast with the neck's upper joint the majority of neck movements are based on rotations when turning from one side of the neck to another.

It is crucial to understand that both joints are there and serve distinct functions when we fall in the wrong position within the neck, and how to correct them.

Additionally the two joints are also held together as the other vertebrae down towards the seventh vertebrae through strong capsules, ligaments and muscles. Between each joint, there is a disc which absorbs shocks when we run, walk and jump, ensuring that any force does not cause damage to the smaller joints which are located in between the vertebrae (facet joint).

The neck's joints

Similar to the thoracic and lumbar spines The neck is supported by muscles. Small muscles of stabilization that connect between vertebrae as well as larger muscles with greater strength that can are more efficient and more forceful moves. Small muscles are known as local muscles, while the larger ones are called global muscles. As I stated in the introduction they work in order to support the neck and moving the neck various directions, and also to move it along with the shoulders to allow us to move in the best and most efficient manner.

The neck's purpose

The main function of the neck is to keep the head upwards. Humans were created with our eyes positioned close in front of our face, similar to the majority of predators found in nature. This is in order to ensure that our gaze stays fixed on our prey, whereas most plant eaters have their eyes positioned further away from the head to make it easier to spot signs of danger.

For us predators who depend heavily in our sight, it's vital to ensure that your head has adequate stability to ensure that it and the muscles are able to keep our head centered on the object. In the present, however, our hunting animals are replaced by computers that puts the same standards for the neck's job. To avoid being injured by a sitting down computer work the purpose of the neck needs to be top-of-the-line. The head must be able to rest at the atlas vertebrae. the muscles local to the spine column need to be able to keep an ideal posture and support the head. At the same at the same time, the global muscles are to be kept in a relaxed state so that they don't get overworked. The main difference in us from our hunter ancestral ancestors is that they were being pushed to the limit by more physical exertion as we spend more time than ever. It doesn't mean, it doesn't mean that the strain on our joints and muscles aren't similar to those of a few thousands of years ago.

Similar to how our eyes are directed in the direction of our prayer, so that we concentrate our eyes at our prayer and pray, we also have the capacity to execute incredible neck movements from all directions, allowing us to detect any dangers either from behind or from the sides. We do not have to turn the entire body to observe what's going on behind us. This means that we have to possess an excellent ability to stabilize the spine column when we move our bodies within the neck to ensure that we don't cause injury to our bodies, however this is not as easy to do!

Mechanisms of injury

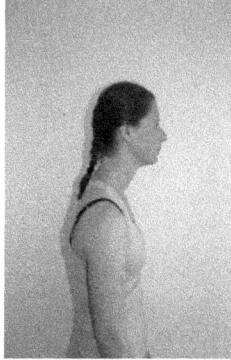

In today's increasingly seated work positions and a growing amount of spending time in our homes The neck isn't able to receive the necessary training to be secure due to its inactivity. Since the body is lazy, and doesn't need to do more work than it is required and doesn't wish to use up energy that is not needed It will adjust to whatever it is exposed to. (See further below).

ı

Image 1: A representation of how the human body adapts to a desk job in which computers are an integral component of everyday life.

Take note of how the lumbar as well as the thoracic spine have been curled and deviated from its normal curvature. When the upper back gets more rounded, it causes cervical vertebrae to follow movements of the spine. However, we do not wish to sit down and stare on the ground. Instead, we raise our heads to keep our eye's view straight forward which is often referred to as"vultures neck" "vultures neck". This happens because the body is trying to ease it for itself, and not spend energy on unnecessary activities even when the task isn't more that "just being sitting!". The major global muscles that use the most energy in the body weaken and the muscles that are less stable rather have to work at higher levels. In the end your posture will remain the same when standing up.

The cinderella Syndrome

As you may have gathered from the story about Cinderella her wicked stepmother always yelled and kept calling for her, and she never had a break.

Cinderella did not get a break every day. Week after week, she was exhausted and exhausted from the laborious work. Similar to Cinderella the muscles of your body work similarly when you sit or standing in a poor place at work, and you notice how it hurts and pull the neck muscles and in the area that is closest to the base of your scull.

What if your muscles could at a rest and not be active longer than they require in the event that your muscles that keep you upright are well-trained and active enough to remain in a comfortable place for longer time? Your muscles wouldn't need to be able to tell you about discomfort but the whole body would be working together.

If you spend a lot of time in front of a screen at job, your body is adjusting to the same task. The smaller muscles in your local area can't maintain your back upright as well as your head into a proper posture. The body will shout for help, and then call on those muscles that are global. The issue lies in the fact that those muscles were specifically designed to perform bigger actions when greater energy is required. They're not built for stabilize your body during tasks that require less power. This can cause an excessive use of the global muscle , which doesn't know how to do its job The only thing it is aware of is that it must be robust. This is why it will do the things it's skilled at, which results in an excessive use.

This is the most common cause for many issues that can arise within the neck. Most commonly, it is the muscles that are big become stressed, the muscles are able to contract, causing blood circulation to slow down because blood can't be moving through the muscle as it is supposed to. The blood cannot supply oxygen to muscles that can cause what's known as ischemic pain (a kind of pain that is caused by an absence of oxygen).

The most commonly used terms used in the clinic

The most frequent problem I experience in a clinic can be described as:

The pain originates from shoulders on one or both sides. It is felt as a band around the skull's base. It is described as a painful area high on the neck. The pain is often described as being sharp and "as like if somebody cut this muscle". Sometimes, headaches can also appearing, sometimes with dizziness. The pain does not disappear completely from paracetamol, but it is alleviated by heating.

AnalyzingThe following is an typical instance from one of the prevalent neck conditions. The majority of the time, it is based on a lot of sitting at the office or at home, or when the patient is standing up with his arms over the shoulders height. Most professions who suffer from this kind of pain such as bus drivers, cleaners, and painters. The static activity of muscles causes them to become to tighten and tense as described previously. The muscle that is overloaded causes pain and is most commonly within the muscle tendons. The muscle most frequently affected is known as musculus in Latin. levitator scapulae. It extends across the upper shoulder to the neck, and connects to the scull's bottom. This muscle is quite tiny and is not able to stand up to a lot of pressure. The muscle is usually stressed and this means it might have to work harder than it needs to. A lot of patients believe they've got an inflammation of the muscles due to the extreme discomfort, but they're just overloaded, without any indication of inflammation.

Treatment-Don't stress about getting treatment for this kind of injury. The fundamental principle is: A muscle that is tight and stressed wants to relax and being activated correctly in the way it was designed to be. It's looking to be contracted and work. You can heal yourself with regular physical exercise such as Nordic walking, using poles in your hands , where you move your shoulders, and stretch the muscle that is tense. The muscles will feel more comfortable and cease to signal discomfort.

In addition to your regular physical exercise that is around 30 minutes per day, you should take breaks if you are working job demands that require you to be seated for long periods of time. Muscles require movement around in order to keep them in good shape and to ensure that blood flow is maintained to the muscles.

Make it a habit of performing these exercises at least once per hour (preferably at least every half an hour) to ensure your muscles are in good shape:

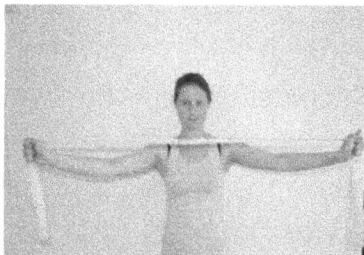

Image 2 This is a workout for the shoulders and neck for people who job or have to work with the body in static positions using their arms or necks.

Performance: Stand straight in the back, then straighten the sternum up, thinking that someone pulls your neck hair into an ideal posture. Maintain your straight arms ahead of you, with your thumbs raised. Make sure that the rubber band is placed over your thumbs, which stimulates the muscles of the rotator-cuff muscles on the shoulder's back effectively. In order to avoid disrupting your neck and your back posture, move your arms straight towards the side and attempt to slow the motion as you return to your front. Repeat this 10-15 times. This improves blood flow and activates muscles that were laying idle. Certain muscles might have started to draw their muscle fibers closer. Then repeat the exercise for another hour!

Examine your neck

In this case, using a few steps that you can take, you'll be able to examine your neck.

Then, we'll discuss how you handle the issues you discover. Ask someone to capture a picture of you from the side while you relax and stand as if you're talking to someone. Then , you can examine your posture in the photo.

Begin by taking a look at your posture and thoracic spine. Are you bending it like it should be or is it bent to much? Take a closer look at the neck. Does the vertical line run over the ear and across the shoulder joint or perhaps the shoulders are just in front of this vertical line? Take a look at the image below, and you'll know the meaning of what I'm saying!

The most frequent issue I observe occurs when the head has been shifted forward to the vertical line as well as the shoulders. This is referred to in the popular jargon of "vultures neck" in common terms. Are you suffering from the neck of a vulture? Verify that the vertical line is just a little behind the top of the ear especially if you look at the rest of your body. The picture at the beginning illustrates an image where the person is mimicking the neck of a vulture. It shows forward head posture as well as rounded shoulders. an "collapsed" the thoracic spine. So 3/3 of errors require correction!

Treatment

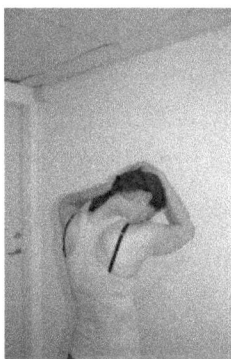

Correcting this kind of bad posture in the shoulder and neck is quite easy. It is important to remember that the majority of "malfunctions" typically occur due to the fact that the body's foundation isn't correct. In this instance, it is the upper back is at fault. The neck is resting on the back of the upper part and the shoulders rest on the sides of it. If the back's upper portion has an overly curvature to the forward (kyphosis) and the cervical and shoulder muscles will follow along with the movements of the thoracic spine upwards. Then, try placing two fingers on your sternum , and move your entire chest towards the sky. Imagine that you're in the military, and the captain tells you to stay straight! This is exactly the kind of motion we'd like to attain. Now , take a photo of yourself in this position. Do you see how shoulders are now relocated backwards? Also, the head is no longer the shoulder area and the neck of the vultures is gone. Also , note how the line vertical is in the right direction and is straight across the top of the ear and to the side and back of the body. This is how it should appear. Great job!

Image 3: Stretching the muscles that are located at the base of the scull. This is a set of muscles situated under the scull's base. As you're in an upward position of your neck (Vultures neck) which causes these muscles to contract since they are required to be working extra hard for keeping your head elevated in the neck's upper joint, so that you keep your eyes on straight ahead.

The neck muscles can be stretched by sitting straight on your back. Place one hand and place it on the side of your head, and slowly lower the neck with the fingers till you notice the first spine process beneath the scull's bottom. Maintain two fingers in that position and hold the process steady. Then, take the hand, and then over your head, then switch to the hand, and grasp your fingers just below the scull's base (as as if you were trying to maneuver your fingers about the field of a football). Bend your head to the side and stretch while moving your hands away. The stretching will be done to your neck muscles. The stretch should last for 30-40 seconds, and repeat the stretch at least a couple of times during the day.

Discussion

As you've seen that it is easy to fall into the position that causes you to shift body parts out of their normal position because of an unintentional displacement of the body's base , which is the thoracic spine. It's also very easy to rectify by bringing your sternum up approximately one inch. This doesn't require a lot of effort or muscle power, however it's crucial to keep reminding yourself to do it. If you're sitting in front of your computer for long periods at work, you've lost the habit of keeping your chest upright and quickly sink back down. There are some strategies that you can employ to keep yourself on track.

1. Set a signal alarm for your cell phone, which will beep every half hour or every hour.

2. Do this each moment you feel like sinking to sit up straight, but also place two fingers to your sternum and raise them while you pay attention to your body. This creates a connection to the brain in a matter of minutes. If you keep doing this over some time and you'll soon

not need to set the alarm on your smartphone and you've established a link between your body and your brain that handles the task on its own. Smart huh!

Chapter 3: What To Consider Prior To Launching A Stretching Program

It's vital to complete these steps prior to beginning your stretching routine. Although starting a regular stretching routine might seem like a simple task, if you're not well-trained, you're more at risk of injuries. It is also helpful to understand what you're doing and help you stick to the plan you select.

Talk with your doctor

Most important you can do prior to beginning the process of stretching is to speak with your physician about your health condition. The doctor will identify the areas you must focus on and the amount you should stretch in order to increase your health in a safe way. If you're experiencing problems with your heart or bones it is possible to start by taking supplements or medicines too.

Find a trainer

If you're not familiar with stretching, or if your doctor suggests that you train with someone to concentrate on specific areas and you'll have to locate a teacher. You might be able to join the classes or contact someone through the local gym for general assistance with stretching.

If you have physical disabilities you might have to locate physical therapists to help.

Locate an Address

It is recommended that you find the best location to perform stretching exercises at the most ease and efficiency. In your home, in an exercise facility or even at your community center, you are able to practice this. Because certain stretches require additional equipment, you'll have to ensure that wherever you go accessible to these. A lot of community centers offer small fitness facilities which are perfect for exercising and generally cheaper than gyms.

Wear appropriate clothing

Dressing in the right way will help you stretch more easily however it doesn't have to be expensive or extravagant Don't stress about it. Just make sure you wear clothes that do not restrict your movement. This could be tight-fitting clothing such as spandex or yoga pants If that's more your style, it's also possible to wear loose-fitting sweatpants.

Find some stretching equipment

If you don't have equipment, you can perform a variety of stretches, however having a few basic pieces of equipment can help you do some of them easier and safer for an older body. Bands for stretching or resistance are ideal to help you intensify and facilitate various stretches.

For various leg exercises An incline board can provide the user with an angle and yoga mats are the ideal way to help cushion your body as you stretch off the ground.

Additionally, there are several different equipment specifically designed to stretch. They are an excellent method to begin since they require you to perform the stretch correctly, which can help prevent injury and enhance the stretch's efficiency.

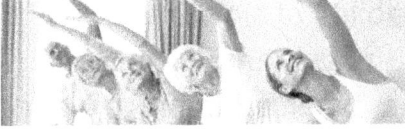

However, they are usually rather expensive however, so when you can find an exercise facility that offers them, that's an ideal alternative.

Once you've put everything in order all you have to do is continue studying to get more information about stretching and begin to stretch each day.

Chapter 4: Utilizing Somatics To Enhance The Flexibility, Posture And Movement Of The Body

The capability of simple exercises that help recover movement in muscles that are painful as well as improve your posture and flexibility is inextricably linked to the capability of your brain's ability to be changed. The relearning of muscle movements is based on the idea that the body needs to be repaired from within; the majority of modern medical treatments focus on treating your body by treating it from outside inside. In contrast to other treatments for injuries to muscles and pains in the body, the somatics approach is not confined by the time. The injury you suffer from could be day old or the past. The exercises will function in the same manner regardless of your age or physical state. Each workout is designed to help your brain to learn how to utilize your muscles correctly.

Somatics can be a good alternative for those who suffers from a lack of flexibility, mobility or poor posture. No matter your age or your lifestyle, you can benefit from these simple and efficient exercises. While the results may not be immediate, they will be evident within a couple of months and will last for a long time and are more effective than many othertraditional types of treatment. Massages, chiropractors, and even prescription medications provide only short-term effects. Learning to use your muscles can have a long-lasting result.

Somatics is actually a great relationship with Yin Yoga, where the exercises are all built around breathing and slow moves. A majority of the poses don't require a lot of balance and physical force. Yin Yoga focuses on slowing the body, just like somatics. This is why it's the perfect option for everyone regardless of age or fitness level.

In actual fact it is true that each of Yin Yoga and somatics are focused on restoring the balance in your own body. As so there's no improper way to do any exercise, as long as you are paying attention to your own inner voice and are focusing on your body's movement. In reality, somatics could help people improve their yin or the yang (the more traditional form of) yoga. It is because they help you break each muscle into smaller pieces and manage each one in turn. If you're able to perform this, even the most complicated of yoga poses is the case of doing each muscle one at a moment with a pre-determined sequence and then watching the exercise work perfectly.

The most important thing about somatics is that it is the most qualified person to teach yourself. You are aware of what parts of your body are in pain or restricted mobility and are the most qualified to be aware of what you are able and should not endure. An instructor who is certified will confirm this, and will focus on your self-awareness. This will enable you to remain in contact with your body, and learn the best postures and exercises for your individual requirements. Much more than any other kind therapy, the one is extremely personal. There are many treatments that emphasize self-awareness and healing the body's inner self However, the majority of alternatives, like the Ortho-Bionomy method, Pilates, Yoga and Continuum aren't as simple to perform at home. They also tend to be more physically demanding.

Exercises that stimulate the muscles can eliminate bad habits in your muscles that cause the lack of movement, and enhance your flexibility. This is because every exercises are intended to stretch your muscle first, then relax it. Your brain is aware of the way that your muscles can be utilized however the body is also using the muscle to the fullest extent. The continual stretching and relaxation does not just relieve tension from your muscles but also allows muscles and joints that surround the muscles to relax and stretch. In the end, all of your body return to their proper positions instead of where they've been moving in the past due to poor posture.

This will lead to an increased mobility and also an increase in flexibility. As your muscles return to normal positions. The body is capable of twisting and bending in ways it hasn't done over the years, but was always capable of. Alongside this increased mobility and flexibility, your posture is likely to improve over time as your internal and external structures as well as muscles are restored to the postures they are supposed to be in. You'll stand higher and perform better. It is possible to follow some guidelines or suggestions on the right posture to adopt to ensure that you don't fall in bad patterns. Concentrating on your posture, movements and flexibility , will make sure you develop habituality to be able to make the right decisions within your body after the second time around. If you practice a good posture and keep repeating it over and over the body will naturally ensure you will maintain the same posture over time. If you are patient and consistent, you will be rewarded by a lifetime of excellent posture, flexibility, and flexibility.

If you're currently experiencing any type of discomfort or pain or if you're likely to experience it in the future, you should try somatics as well as some of the exercises they offer to avoid issues that could affect your joints, muscles or tendons in the near future. Somatics is an important way to go for anyone. the ability to manage your muscles on an individual basis and maintain your posture when doing so is an achievement that anyone can appreciate. Learn the somatic movements covered in this book, and begin your journey to relief from a variety of issues with movement or problems with flexibility, as well as bad posture. It's very simple to start and the results will be evident very quickly.

Chapter 5: Pranayama

Pranayama comes from the two Sanskrit words 'prana' which is a synonym for vital energy, and 'ayama' meaning control. In a literal sense, pranayama is the control the vital force within you. It is however more often interpreted as control of breath as it is in yoga philosophy. It is usually associated as 'vital energy' or the vital force.

The techniques used in pranayama operate by assuming that breathing can be controlled to adhere to specific rhythms. This can allow you to relax or concentrate your mind and body. Additionally, by learning how to breathe properly, pranayama also claims you will increase your general health and energy levels.

To put it in a more precise manner it is believed that pranayama does not just to aid in weight loss but also help cleanse the blood, eliminate the toxins, increase concentration and clarity, boost our threshold for pain and reduce the feeling of pain, and help us feel calm and relaxed. There is no shortage of advantages!

Depending on the material you are using it is possible to find dozens of different methods for pranayama. Certain types of yoga connect prana to energy and link it with particular body parts that are similar to chakras. The yogi's mental energy or emotion is merely a kind of prana. All the different types of prana are derived from breath.

In addition, the breath influences the way that prana flows within the body. Rapid, fast breathing can result in flashes of energy while slow, rhythmic breathing produces continuous, constant energy flows. The different energy flows affect our mental state with slower breathing resulting in calm and steady state of mind.

Similar to how, as time passes, these breathing patterns and energy flow affect the body. Breathing that is constrictive and short-lived causes harm to your body over time, and could cause fatigue and sickness. However, deep, efficient breathing increases your body's energy, making you more durable and long-lasting. Then, these changes in your body caused by the breath is thought to impact our character. A tense breathing pattern can cause anxiety; peaceful breathing is the key to a relaxed mind.

In the ancient texts prana was believed to flow through and coalesce into small areas of the body known as nadis according to some writings, there are as high as 72,000 nadis within the body. Today, the movement of prana throughout the body has been linked to the nerve system as well as the transfer of power from the spinal cord and brain to all the small branches of the nerves across the body.

The goal of pranayama is to shift the breath to come from the navel and the bottom of the spine, not the chest's nostrils. While you don't have to be a believer in the spiritual theories that the ancient yogis believed in, it is believed that breathing in this way can increase the energy flow in the root chakra, which, in turn, can aid and bring about a higher spiritual awakening.

In the same way, pranayama is thought to be a part in Raja yoga, also known as royal yoga, which focuses on the more spiritual and esoteric aspect of yoga. A lot of westerners have embraced these methods to reduce stress, fight depression and enhance their overall happiness with their lives.

The most fundamental stage of pranayama is to concentrate on breathing. This form of practice is the basis of many spiritual and religious practices found in the East. By focusing constantly on breathing your mind and concentration are honed and enhanced, which could be the basis for higher levels and more advanced forms of meditation.

For the first time, you must sit in a comfortable place in a space free of distractions. It is ideal if this is a space that you rarely spend a lot of time in, and it is not cluttered with your normal mental associations and routines. Ideally, you'll place yourself in the half-lotus or the perfect posture, in which your feet rest against the lower thigh area of your opposite leg. If this is too painful and uncomfortable for your needs standing or kneeling in other positions can suffice.

The goal of focusing on breathing is to improve diaphragmatic breathing. The diaphragm muscle is located beneath the lungs that expands and contracts as you breathe. A deeper breathing pattern is linked to more diaphragm motion while the breath that is shallow is linked to the shoulders and chest.

According to yoga, there are three kinds of breathing: diaphragmic breathing which originates around the belly button breathing, Thoracic breathing (mid-chest) and the clavicular breathing (upper chest). The majority of these types of breathing are referred to by naming them deep, medium, and shallow breathing, respectively.

Deep breathing is believed as the best effective. Breathing shallowly can happen in the course of exercise, but it can also happen in cases where breathing has been damaged due to asthma or smoking. The moderate breathing is the most common breathing method for the majority of people. Based on the knowledge that breathing has an impact on our well-being, mood and our personality, it could be concluded that you could, in a way, enhance our lives by learning how to breathe deeply.

For deep breathing exercises Simply breathe through your nose. But make sure to breathe at a slow pace. It is believed that you breathe about 15-20 times every minute. According to pranayama experts it is recommended that you are able to breathe more than this.

While you breathe, rest your hands on your stomach (diaphragm). As you breathe, your diaphragm will be stretched out and should shrink when you exhale. If you're struggling to breathe deeply then try to rid your lungs first. Breathe as deeply as that you can, and then take some time before breathing backwards. The next breath will be more deep and will come from your belly.

In particular, if you're trying to breathe more slowly it is best specifically to breathe more slowly. It is believed that by when you allow air to fill and remain in your lungs for longer you increase the amount of oxygen that your body absorbs and also boost metabolism.

An advanced technique for pranayama involves putting a weight on your belly while you relax and breathe. This will strengthen the diaphragm as well as increase the benefits of pranayama practice even more.

Furthermore, it is believed that pauses in breathing between exhalation and inhalation may be beneficial. Make sure to allow a 1 to 2 second interval between exhalation and inhalation however, do not feel lightheaded if this is uncomfortable for you.

If you are a beginner, this is all you have to do. It seems simple however, once you've attempted to keep your breathing in check for a prolonged amount of time you will be able to see that it's quite difficult. The mind is naturally inclined to tendency to wander, and deep anxieties and tensions come in. If you experience this attempt to keep going.

Stress can be uncomfortable, and your mind naturally has the habit of fleeing and distracting its thoughts. Do not allow it! Just feel your anxiety or stress in its subtle magnitude and force. While it might take some time but as you continue to take a deep breath, these emotions will diminish and dissipate. It's not possible to conquer stress by doing this, but you let it to flow and disappear eventually becoming peaceful and serene.

Chapter 6: Experiments For The Advanced

The exercises that are more advanced can assist to maintain an upright head position. After pain levels have diminished and you are able to complete the following strengthening exercises can help promote good posture. Incorporating them into your workout routine, and in the case of transverse abdominal exercises, in daily activities will lower the chance of developing injuries due to postural problems.

Shoulder Flexion in the direction of the Wall

This is a variation using the postural muscles in the mid-back.

Instructions:

1. Lean back with your shoulders against the wall.

2. Make sure you press your shoulder blades downwards and then up against the wall.

3. Keep your arms straight and gradually raise your arms until you reach the level of your shoulders straight ahead.

4. Slowly lower to return to the starting point.

5. Do 10 repetitions, which is enough for three sets.

Tips:

Maintain Your back to the wall during the exercise.

* When lifting the arms to shoulder height, make sure to point your thumbs upwards. This will prevent shoulder impingement.

* To build up your fitness, you can add an additional dumbbell to each hand.

Chin Tuck and Shoulder Flexion

This variation in exercise offers an arduous challenge that can help maintain and keep improving muscle strength in the neck's deep flexor muscles. After pain levels have reduced or eliminated, adding this workout into your weekly routine can prevent your the recurring neck pain that is common to desk workers.

Instructions:

1. Begin on all fours by placing your hands directly beneath your shoulders, and your knees directly beneath your hips.

2. Adjust the shoulder blades by squeezing the shoulder blades down and into.

3. Maintaining a straight and neutral spine, gradually lower the chin.

4. In the same way you should bring your arm straight ahead.

5. Relax the chin slowly and then lower the arm to where it was before.

6. Repeat on the other side.

7. Do 10 repetitions over 3 sets.

Tips:

* Be sure to gently bend your neck as much as you can comfortably.

Continue to squeeze the shoulder blades as you lift one arm. Don't rotate the trunk. The spine and the trunk must remain stable and neutral.

* If you are performing this exercise it is recommended that it is recommended

that the TA exercise below could be added to ensure that a neutral back is kept.

Exercises for the Transverse Abdominal

As we've mentioned before all body parts is interconnected. Postural problems in the upper back can impact the lower area and reverse. The transverse abdominal muscles, or muscles of the TA are deeper abdominal muscles. They function as a girdle that protects and supporting the lower the pelvic and back. Even the best athlete may have weak TA muscle. They are often overlooked and instead, a lot of people concentrate on the'six-pack abdominal muscles.

The TA muscles are the primary focus of many low back rehabilitation programs. Making sure the lower part of the trunk is properly supported will help to improve the overall health of your spine. While it's not specifically an advanced exercise and is not required to correct the forward posture of the head It is an essential muscle that must be trained to promote the proper alignment of the spine. It is a given that everyone should learn to stretch the muscles of the TA. It will save you many visits to the doctor or physical therapists, and could prevent painful episodes that are caused by low back pain, which can result in the onset of a number of other ailments. The most basic steps for how to engage the TA muscle are given below, and are followed by suggested steps.

Instructions:

1. Relax on your back while keeping your knees bent. Keep your feet are flat.

2. To engage the TA muscles imagine a rope that is pulling your hip bones in a row or stopping your urine flow.

3. Keep the contraction going to 5-10 seconds.

4. Do 10 repetitions, which is enough for 3 sets.

Tips:

* Be sure to breathe through the exercise. Do not hold your breath.

* You should keep your back on the floor or in bed during the workout.

* To advance in this workout, you must follow these steps below.

Progression One:

Instructions:

1. Lay on your back by bending your knees, and feet are flat.

2. To tighten the TA muscles, visualize a rope pulling your hip bones in a row or stopping your urine flow.

3. Keep the contraction in place and keep that leg in a bent position, then slowly raise one leg.

4. Do not stop for more than 3-5 seconds.

5. Lower the leg until it is back to its starting position. Repeat the process on both sides.

6. Do 10 repetitions, which is enough for three sets.

Tips:

* Be sure to breathe through the exercise. Don't hold your breath.

Your back must remain on the floor or in bed during the exercise.

• Reset your contraction intervals between repetitions to make sure that you don't begin to use the back muscles.

Progression Two:

Instructions:

1. Relax on your back while keeping your knees bent. Keep your feet straight.

2. To engage the TA muscles imagine a rope pulling your hip bones in a row or stopping your urine flow.

3. Maintain the contraction while keeping the knees bent. Slowly raise one leg.

4. Slowly lift the other leg.

5. For 2-5 seconds, hold the button.

6. Slowly lower one foot to begin, and then lower another leg.

7. Do 10 repetitions over three sets.

Tips:

* Be sure to breath throughout your exercise. Don't hold your breath.

* Keep your back on the bed or floor during the workout.

• Reset your contraction every repetition, to make sure that you don't begin to use the back muscles.

If you are beginning to feel pain on your back you can try mixing Progression One with Progression Two. In other words, try Progression Two for 1-2 sets followed by Progression One for 1-2 sets. In total, the number of set must be 3 when you combine them. Choose the one that works and feels most comfortable.

Progression Three:

Instructions:

1. Relax on your back by bending your knees, and feet are flat.

2. To tighten the TA muscles, imagine a rope pulling your hip bones to stop in the urine stream.

3. Make sure to hold the contraction. Lift your feet just 1 inch above the mat or bed.

4. With your feet just slightly above the bed or mat and gradually move one foot upwards.

5. Keep it for two seconds.

6. Slowly lower the leg and repeat the process on both sides.

7. Do 10 repetitions, which is enough for 3 sets.

Tips:

Make sure you breath throughout your exercise. Don't hold your breath.

* Keep your back on the floor or in bed during the workout.

• Reset your contraction intervals between repetitions to make sure that you do not begin using the back muscles.

If you start to feel pain on your back consider mixing Progression Two with Progression Three. In other words, try Progression Three for 1-2 sets before doing Progression Two for 1-2 sets. Total number of sets must be three when they are combined. Pick the set that is most effective and feels most comfortable.

* To continue you can go through Progression Three, but with both legs extended at simultaneously.

The opening to the Thoracic Region

In the previous section of this book Thoracic outlet syndrome can be an adverse effect that can result from an inclination of the head that is forward. In addition, breathing difficulties and other problems could occur. A foam roller can aid in opening the chest and stopping the forward downward sagging into the shoulder. This exercise is great for maintaining and to incorporate into your routine after your pain has diminished and the prevention of future recurrences is the objective.

Instructions:

1. Lay on your back by bending your knees. Keep your feet flat. lay a foam roller along the vertical spine line.

2. Reach your arms out towards the sides, keeping your palms up.

3. Maintain this position for 30 seconds to one minute and one-half. Do this 2-3 times a every day or in conjunction with your regular exercise routine.

Tips:

* Make sure you breath throughout your exercise. Don't hold your breath.

Relax your neck and rest it against the foam roller or pile of pillows to provide support. Don't allow your neck to hang awkwardly from the roller's edge.

* Try to hold the position for the position for as long as you can. It should feel comfortable stretching your chest. Also, you may feel a soft stretch across your chest muscles as they are stretched.

Chapter 7: The 8 Types Of A Posture That Is Off

A majority of people be afflicted by some form of pain throughout their lives. It doesn't matter whether they work 5 days a week, or just one day per week, they'll experience pains, believe it or it's not. The discomfort could be caused by aging or an absence of physical exercise. Gravity could be a factor in the discomfort.

Like I've stated that, every single one of us could suffer from pain that is severe in our lives, provided we take the appropriate precautions to avoid these. You must keep an eye on the various types of bad postures , and how bad postures may result in deterioration in the event that we don't take proper into consideration the care they require.

In this chapter, we're going to talk about the 8 types of poor posture.

1. KYPHOSIS

This is a rare condition caused by the upward sloping of the back.

What does it look like

Kyphosis is visible on both sides your body, particularly when bent towards the front or when standing upright. If you have shoulders that are rounded it is possible to observe a rounded curve around your waist. (You'll notice the curve more in bending).

If you look at our body it will be apparent that the spine in the back is designed to be straight line. The spine is comprised of two curvatures, kyphotic and lordotic, that create an S-Shape. Both curves attempt to be balanced. While standing, you must make sure you are aligned according to the effects of kyphosis. Kyphosis is when the shoulders turn rounder, typically in the 20o to 40o range. between 40 and 20o.

How do I detect

The first step in identifying Kyphosis is to undergo physical therapy. The aim of the physical therapy is to find out if the curvature increases in time. If not, the exercises contained in this book can greatly assist to strengthen the muscles of the spine. If physical therapy results not, then you'll have to do core muscle strengthening exercises.

Kyphosis is treatable without surgery.

It may circulate and move towards the back of the middle and lower back.

2. ROUNDED SHOULDERS

What does it look like

Rounded shoulders is a term that refers to the appearance of shoulders placed further forward than the typical. Usually, rounded shoulders are associated with a forward posture that can increase the tilt of the thoracic kyphosis.

How to Find

A way to spot the appearance of rounded shoulders is by standing in the mirror and let your arms appear to protrude at your sides. If your numbs point towards the front, it indicates you've got a weak back and a tense chest giving the impression that you have rounded shoulders.

The rounded shoulders are not a condition that could be treated, but it can cause is a stern reminder of your daily activities. Therefore, if you fix your shoulders' roundedness today and then return to your old habits, and do not bother to perform any exercises in the future The rounded shoulders are likely to return.

You should set aside minimum 30 minutes every day to do the exercises. You don't require these exercises every day. Just performing them once or twice every week, will help you in rehabilitating this posture.

3. LORDOSIS

What does it look like

Lordosis can be caused by the natural curve that occurs in lower back. The curvature occurs when the body is in an extended curve around the stomach which causes it to protrude. It also causes the pelvis curve upwards and down. Lordosis can make you appear to have swaybacks and causes the buttocks to appear more noticeable.

How do you detect

Lordosis can be identified by anyone. It is easy to detect it by lying on a flat surface and looking at how much space is between your body and floor. It will be obvious that you've Lordosis If you discover that you are able to put fingers between the back of your body and floor.

Lordosis doesn't constitute a major condition that requires extensive medical attention. It's the curvature that is located around the back. The proper posture of lordosis can help support the weight of your head. A proper posture for Lordosis can also allow you to bend and move by flexing your head and aligning it over your pelvis. The exercises that follow in the following section will help reverse lordosis in the event that you find that your back returns to its normal posture when standing straight. However, if you notice that your back doesn't change when you stand straight, then you have consult with your physician regarding the procedure.

4. SWAYBACK

What does it look like

The first thing you need to know regarding swayback concerns that the pelvis (the pelvis is the region of the spine that is above the legs and is below). The optimal posture helps support the normal lordosis that is found in the back of your lower back. The arch, or s-curve, helps balance all the skeletal components of the body. They collaborate to assist in supporting the body weight.

Therefore, the spine compensates and the curves of the mid and upper bodies increase. The most significant movement in the swayback position is the movement backwards that the spine of the thoracic.

Swayback happens when the back arch is bent in such a manner that the pelvis stays in a forward-facing position.

How do you recognize

The first step to determine if you suffer from swayback is to examine your body from both areas of your back. It is possible to ask a friend to take photos of your body looking from the side. What you'll want to see is your shoulders.

If your shoulders are placed in a vertical line to the hips that means you're in good posture. However, if your shoulders are in front of the hips, you are in the swingback.

You must make sure the shoulders of both are in the back. If both shoulders appear as if they're currently behind the hip, then there is the possibility of swingback. Another method to recognize swayback, and make up for the upper back tilting back. This is to fall on your head whenever you stand or attempt to walk.

The only way that your body is able to attempt to find balance is to move your head backwards and give the appearance of a Hunchback posture, which is also called Kyphosis. If you're experiencing this and you are an swingback.

In this case I've provided a few easy exercises that you can adhere to.

If you suffer from any kind of postural disorder this deformity can cause the spine adapt to one region, to compensate any imbalance due to the deformity.

People who have swayback tend to place greater weight onto their feet instead of their heels. Swaybacks can make you appear like you have an oomph belly, even though you don't actually have. Many of my patients I've treated have pains when they sit for an extended period of time. They must always stretch their bodies outwards without realizing they're harming their disc.

5. FORWARD HEAD POSTURE

The postural issue is due to poor habits that have been accumulated for a considerable period of period of. Through many years, I've helped numerous patients suffering from shoulder pain and headaches. In the majority of cases I've found that they are suffering from an forward-facing head position.

What does it look like

Forward head posture is when you're placing on your head the burden onto your body in front of you, causing muscles have to be working more. Head posture that is forward is among the most frequent causes of neck discomfort.

How do you recognize

Put your back to the wall, and just six inches from the wall.

Take note of how many fingers can put between the back of your neck , and on the wall. If you are able to put three fingers on the neck's back then you're in a an forward posture for your head. In this situation your muscles and shoulder joints start to weaken.

A forward head position can put stress on the tissues, which could result in the shoulders being rounded. This doesn't stop there, it also puts a tremendous amount of stress on the neck as well as the shoulders.

Additionally, the forward posture of the head can affect your center of gravity for the entire body.

6. UNEVEN SHOULDERS

What is it that it appears to look like?

If someone claims that they have shoulders that are uneven is a sign that their shoulders are towards the front, and one shoulder has a higher level than their other. For example, if you take a look at your shoulders when carrying a large bag of weight on your shoulders, you'll see that one of your shoulders will slump to support the shoulder of the other. Uneven shoulders begin with one area of the body and goes on until it is expanded to other body parts.

How do you recognize

The most effective way to identify irregular shoulders is to examine and observe which shoulder has a higher level than your other. It is easy to do this yourself by using an mirror.

7. FUNCTIONAL (NON-STRUCTURAL) SCOLIOSIS

(An important aspect to be aware of the exercises in this publication deal with functional Scoliosis, not structural. The difference between these two cases is the fact that both is able to be addressed with the exercises included in this publication.)

What is it that it appears to look like?

It happens when the spine takes on a curved position. When we consider functional scoliosis, it is considering scoliosis that could be fixed or corrected. There are two kinds of functional scoliosis, structural scoliosis and non-structural (functional) Scoliosis.

The issue we'll be examining is the one that functions. The functional one could be caused by various reasons. It could be due to the tension in the muscles where there's one muscle which is pulling tight or towards the other direction, or it may suffer from muscle spasms in which muscles don't contract, causing curvature of the spine. If you're considering the scoliosis, you're seeing a spinal column which is straight forward away from the centerline.

How can you tell

To identify if you've got scoliosis, you must have someone examine your spine from the back. If there is a curvature that is not straight on your spine, it is likely that you are suffering from Scoliosis. To determine if your Scoliosis can be classified as functional (non-structural) it is necessary to straighten your spine. If your spine's curvature increases, you are suffering from functional Scoliosis.

8. FLATBACK

Flatback syndrome is a condition that affects the lower back or lumbar spine. Flatback can cause an inclination of moderately on the back. If the upper spines flatten out completely, there is an increase in the flatness of it that could cause pain with the back of your lower and the hips, throughout the neck and spine.

How do you recognize

One of the first tests to determine if you've got flatbacks is to take the side view. Keep your posture as normal. Do not try to move your body in any way. Check to see whether there's rounding or flattening of the entire spine. If so, then you've got flatback syndrome.

Chapter 8: Strategies To Improve Your Sitting, Standing, Standing, And Sleeping Posture

Standing Posture

Locate your centre. Balance and alignment is the key when it comes to the correct posture for standing. It can lead to a an appearance that is confident. Here are some suggestions to attain the ideal standing posture:

Place your feet shoulder width apart. It is the same position that you use for working out, or for a variety of other activities.

Make sure you stand straight. This is the first step to achieving an ideal standing posture and must be practiced several times. When you begin to develop the right posture it will become routine.

Place your body weight onto the soles of your feet. If you sit in your heels, your normal tendency of your body is to slump. Instead, try standing on the soles of your feet. Then observe the way your body moves as you rock back and make sure you are on your heels. It is vital to notice how your body changes to a slouchy stance in a single movement.

The next step in improving your posture while standing may seem strange initially, but make sure you keep your shoulders straight. It's another way to improve your posture.

Lift your head and then return. Imagine reaching for the roof using you head on top. Place your head on top of your neck and spine when you do it. This will not just improve your posture, but you'll also appear healthier and more slender.

Fix standing position with assistance:

Place your back against the wall or door in a straight line, with the back of your head as well as your shoulders and butt only in front of it. If you feel uncomfortable and uncomfortable but don't fret because once you establish proper posture the body will be able to be taught to not be uncomfortable standing this way.

Walking Posture:

Start by having a good standing position. Standing in a good position is the first step toward walking in a posture that is good. Keep your head upright with your chest up, shoulders back and your the eyes straight ahead. do not push your head forward.

Improve sitting posture:

What are the most frequent times you received this advice from your parents or teachers. For the majority people, the advice was filed under "eat your peas" as well as "your eyes will remain in that manner." However, this is a serious issue to think about. Particularly, today, when the majority of us work at our desks it is crucial to adhere to these guidelines to protect your health and your posture. If you sit at a desk for extended hours and have the option of a chair, choose one that's specifically designed to provide proper support, and is specifically designed to accommodate your height and weight. You could also utilize a small cushion for back support if you don't have the alternative. Adjust your back to the back of your office chair. It will stop you from sitting too far forward or slumping, since this is something you might do after sitting for too much at your workstation.

For standing posture it is important to keep your shoulders square and straight with your head straight, as well as your collar bones as well as your back and feet in alignment. Do a simple two-step desk routine to correct your posture.

Make sure your feet are on the ground or in a footrest (incase your legs aren't reaching the to the ground).

Adjust your position and chair to ensure that your arms aren't straight, but bent. Try to achieve 75-90 degrees angle between your elbows. Keep in mind that if they're too straight, you're sitting too far back however if they're greater that 90 degrees it indicates that you're in a position that is too close, or you're just slouching.

Take standing breaks:

If you believe you're sitting in a perfect position, when you're in one of the priciest chairs you can find (although the cost of the chair has nothing to do with have anything to do with comfort in this instance) you must get up and stretch or do some walking, exercise or simply stand for a while. Your body was not meant to sit all daylong, and a number of recent studies have revealed that sitting for an extended period of time can be a trigger for numerous diseases and ailments. So, keep moving!

How to drive:

The importance of good posture is not just suggested for better posture however, it is also essential for safety-related issues that are more practical. The car's protective and seating systems were created to ensure that you sit in your correct position, and could be a factor in safety in the event of a crash.

Make sure you keep your back against the seat and your head resting against the headrest.

Make sure your seat is at the proper distance between the pedal and steering wheel. If you're leaning forward, trying to reach for the wheel, or even pointing your toes at the wheel, you're far from the wheel. Also, if you're in a tangle with your chin resting on the wheel, that means you're not far enough away.

Set the height of the rest It is essential that the head rest you have is correctly adjusted. Turn the head rest around according to your needs, so as to keep a distance of not more than 4 inches (10cm) between your head's back and the rest of your head.

Pose for sleeping

Sleep well: You may not always keep a good posture when you sleep, but there are ways to improve your posture. If you choose a mattress with a firmer surface to ensure the proper support for your back. If you sleep on your back, it can help keep your shoulders straight and it's generally easier on your spine when compared to sleeping on your stomach.

If you prefer sleeping on your back then you can add an extra cushion between your knees. it can help keep your spine straight and aligned.

Use a pillow to ensure an appropriate alignment and support for the head and shoulders. Do not over-use the pillows as it could cause your head to be bent in an awkward position. This can cause damage to your posture and leave you up stiff, sore and fatigued.

Chapter 9: What Causes Us To Have Posture Problems?

What is the reason we experience lower Back Pain?

While our posture can be an excellent place to begin when looking at back pain Research has shown that stress can be the main cause for the vast majority of people of back pain. However, you may notice that back pain becomes more severe in certain circumstances like sitting at the desk for prolonged times. It is crucial to be aware of the time when your back pain becomes more noticeable, and then simply look at what you've been doing the past couple of hours.

"BEGIN to write down notes whenever you notice your back pain being particularly strong. Be aware of what you're doing and what you've been doing for the past few hours prior to this. AFTER A FEW TIMES OF DOING THIS, OBSERVE WHETHER THERE ARE ANY PATTERNS TO WHEN YOUR BACK PAIN IS WORSE"

Regarding posture and back pain in particular the way we sit can be a major factor. In general, if we're lying in a slumped or slouchy position with no adequate support for our lower back it can result in back pain in the future. Slumping down in a chair can be more comfortable than sitting upright initially because it seems like it's taking the muscles to exert less and as time passes, our bodies get is accustomed to this posture and automatically adopts it as our preferred sitting posture. But over time, the slumped posture can put an additional strain on muscles as well as soft tissues in our lower back. This can result in tension that could cause pain later in the future. We'll be looking at the best way to sit at a later time in our book, and how we can help support our backs properly and release this tension on our muscles.

What causes us to experience neck as well as Shoulder Pain?

The constant usage of laptops, computers as well as mobile phones, among other everyday activities may create tension and pain in our shoulders and necks. When we sit in a hunched position over laptops, for instance, we usually put more stress on our lower backs which results in lower back pain and a weaker upper. The chest also gets tighter because of the hunched-up position which causes an increase in tension in the chest region, which could result in a strain on neck and shoulders. It is also possible to develop problems with our neck like putting our chin forward of our body , instead of straight and in line to our spinal column. Also, we may turn our shoulders in lieu or pulling them forward, tightening the chest , but not using our muscles of the upper back. All of these could cause problems with our shoulders, chest neck, and neck as well as things like headaches.

What causes us to feel pain in our Hips, Legs and Feet?

While most posture problems can affect any part of the body but some have more particularities than other. Our foot position and bad walking habits can impact our knees, pelvis and feet, which can cause discomfort and tension in these locations. Because of our habits when walking many of us tend to walk with our buttocks dangling out too much while our hips are sinking and glute muscles that haven't being properly used when walking. These could cause problems within the lower body and also in those in the upper. As with many of these problems they can be difficult to recognize at first because they're something we've done for all of the time, it could seem as normal.

The way our feet are placed when we stand can create imbalances that run through the spine and across the body. If your feet aren't aligned correctly this can affect everything else. The most commonly encountered issue in the feet area is called "duck feet" which is when your toes and feet point inwards diagonally when standing, instead of being straight towards you. Additionally, the way we place our feet on the floor can cause issues. If we tend to put our weight on the inner side of our feet instead of being evenly distributed throughout feet, it is possible that we might suffer from imbalances in our spine and legs. This is often caused by the types of shoes we choose to wear or our poor walking habits learned over time. We do not think the possibility that our actions might not be the most healthy method of doing something because it's familiar to us.

Chapter 10: The Specific Motion Of Man

The specific man's motion can be defined as the collection of energy, dynamic, and information-related events that are convergent in the bipedal ambulation that alternates (motion with progress) as well as in the upright station (motion with no progression).

Of the various structures in the brain and central nervous system over a quarter of them participate directly and over half are involved indirectly in the design and execution of motions; the man who has muscles of 650 and bones of is the most fundamentally an "motor creature."

Man must move for his well-being and survival. being. Because of this, locomotion is the one that has the highest priority over all other activities. Actually, in the realm of life at the top level, locomotion is the unique human movement, which is the most complicated natural process. The notion that the intellect is the only thing that separates man has been largely discredited and it is now recognized that they also acknowledge the origin of the brain's activity with the acquisition of the bipod morphomechanical condition, and the release of hands is an additional consequence (Paparella Treccia, 1988). Motor functions as well as the body, viewed in many cultures as subordinate objects and subordinate to cognitive processes and our minds, constitute in fact the basis of the abstract actions that we are proud of as well as the language that is the basis of our mind along with our thought processes. When we are in the embryonic stage in the fetal as well as the early stages of childhood the action precedes sensation and reflexes are performed and then interpreted. It is through sensory reflexes of the proprioceptive that representations (engrams) are created that facilitate the development of more complex motor skills, and similar concepts. When you are in a stressful situation (high stress) the muscular system functions as an extremely important system. When it is activated, other systems, like the ones responsible to perceive feelings as well as attention, cognitive processes and so on. They are in an essentially blocked state and are linked in the subconscious with the performance of vital actions to survive like escape or attack, the search for food, the search for a sexual partner, or the nest. Today we understand that a simple exercise in nature can result in a dramatic rebalancing between brain hemispheres two.

The present human body is, in essence, over all, a result of the need to carry out an efficient and effective walk on two feet within the gravitational field over natural uneven terrain. Based on this theory it is essential for man to move without a lot of energy usage within a continuous gravity field. There is also the added benefit that during the entire journey, all structures (muscles bones, ligaments and tendons, etc.) are exposed to a single minimum stress.

The importance of POSTURE

One of the perhaps the most overlooked aspect of fitness is posture of the person. Certain authors discuss certain books, but the training card is never writtenin reference to a hypothetical model that is theoretically perfect in the back, chest shoulders, arms, abdominals, and legs. This is not the first issue to be considered prior to analyzing the weight, height, and body fat.

The study of posture is totally ignored and the body areas are taught with training cards that emphasize every technique available that include all combinations of exercises taking into consideration thrust and traction as well as all the series/repetition strategies but none of them take into consideration the possibility the person who is required to do it could be in an improper posture, for instance, due to an Kyphosis .

The posture of a person is a signpost to the condition of the skeletal system with respect to the muscles of the subject It isn't just an aesthetic aspect of good posture.

So a posture that is not correct will always indicate a problem with the design that the person is in.

A faulty general arrangement can have consequences for all movements which are carried out and specifically, those that are in the weak region of the postural. This is why exercises designed to strengthen specific muscles, but with the wrong posture, does not actually work, or recruit them in a way that creates a general imbalance.

An example? This is a good one: have been wondering why certain people are more adept at stretching parallel lines? In contrast to bench presses? Since most of the time the subjects, in addition to being light and thin and have a kyphotic body posture with an anteriorly curved and curved shoulder. In this posture, which is usually paired with a chest that is flat, the pectoral muscle is unable to fully extend , and therefore build the strength needed as it works half-way down, but will yield early and then transferring the work to the tricepsmuscles, which is the weakest link in the chain of kinetics for the bench that is used to relieve stress and will give way sooner. This same exercise will perform better than stretching to the parallels as in such a workout the humerus is located adjacent to the trunk makes use of its strength. large pectoralis. It is also a great source of strength for all the pectoralis of the small.

For these people it's pretty sad. They try the bench, but get poor results They try pre-boring, with the same negative results, then they go to the parallels but at the end of the day the pectorals shrink regardless and, if they do, they appear to be "tits." increasing and increasing in posture.

By analyzing the posture first it's better to get rid of all exercises for the pectorals , and the pull-ups using supine grips with a focus on an intense exercise for the back. after the month, these people will be able to display an impressively improved posture and, without having been trained, as well as the overall appearance of their chests and pectorals will improve. Sure, a month is enough time to get an idea of the results but to become a more stable posture, it requires at minimum one year. An incorrect posture does not only impact the pectorals; it also affects the abdominals , legs and the legs, etc. It is so crucial in the training of the bb.

Do you have any questions about why certain individuals, while working their abs through a variety in repetitions, exercises and hundreds appear to have a bulging abdominal?

If other people are doing the squat in a strict manner in a proper manner are complaining about fatigue of lower back muscles that are higher than the quadriceps?

Why do some subjects have large biceps, even when the barbell curls are on?

The reason is generally similar: improper posture, an unbalanced position and a load discharge that is not directly on the muscles of the target rather onto the vertebral or the skeletal structures.

A bad posture negates the advantages of exercises that are designed to work skeletal muscles in accordance to a predetermined direction, and a path that changes when a posture is incorrect. Additionally, the development of muscles that is based on a well-balanced postural subject can take completely different forms in an unbalanced subject, frequently aggravates the problems already existing.

Let's look at how we can determine whether our posture is correct or not.

A postural study, one that naturally, must be confirmed in orthostatic by an orthopedist. It can be carried out using an "do the job yourself" method.

The exercise should be conducted with the help of an individual who, from a distance will first be more impartial than the subject is in general, and later be able to effectively evaluate the posterior and lateral vision that is impossible to confirm by himself.

The study must be performed with an objective examination performed with the aid of a "graduated" reference that is placed in front of the object. The "graduated" references is adequate for walls with tiles or bricks to ensure that the difference of the right body portion in relation towards the left is easily discernible. Plumb lines can also be beneficial to confirm the right-left shift that occurs in scoliosis.

Then, sit down and naked in a comfortable posture, frontal with your arms in front of you and your palms pointing towards your legs, feet slightly separated but in a parallel line. Make sure you don't perform any contraction or extension, retraction or other move that alters your body structure. If you do in a way, you'll be deceiving yourself.

Then we look at the most important elements of posture by doing the frontal, lateral and an analysis of the posterior.

- The frontal examination of shoulder height: If one shoulder is higher than the other then scoliosis may be present.

Hands positioned at a level with the thighs. If the shoulders are not symmetrical, the hands must be slightly different height. However, the difference is concealed by the different extensions of wrists and arms.

An angle that is formed between neck and shoulders If the line connecting the neck with the shoulders creates an angle of more than 90 degrees The shoulders are referred to"Postiglione" or "Postiglione" which is usually coupled with kyphosis and winged scapulas.

The hip level: If the iliac crest of one is higher than the other, scoliosis or shorter or longer length for lower limbs might be present.

Leg line Straight, arcuate or x with respect to the knee as well as to the articulation tibiotarsal joint.

The lateral analysis

The spine's curve at the shoulder level: If the curve of the spine is more than normal, there is a kyphosis or the so-called "hump," it is usually associated with internalized shoulders (forward motion).

The position of the shoulder blades If the lower part of your shoulders (they have triangular bone structures) is visible or"winged" shoulder blades or "winged shoulder blades" are present, and the inability to include the above is not dependent on the thickness of the person.

The spine's curve at the lumbar point The curve that is physiological is more prominent and curved, it is a sign of lordosis as well as accentuated retroversion, or an anteversion.

Analysis of the back :

every aspect of the analysis of the frontal view are valid but connected to the rearview.

The presence of scoliosis will be visible posteriorly through a distinct hypertrophy and contraction of one side in comparison with the opposite. If you consider as a support point to the plumb line the nape's central point or the prominences of seven cervical vertebrae, as well for an escape spot, the intergluteal fold. It will be apparent the movement in the column of vertebrae one side or another when there is scoliosis.

In this moment, I'd affirm that, in a comprehensive manner the most common postural issues identified (scoliosis, Kyphosis, lordosis shoulder blades and anterior shoulders along with "stud" shoulder blades) can lead to problems with developing the pectorals and biceps abdominals, and legs.

This could be the least of all evils. Imagine what might be the consequences for a person suffering from Scoliosis who has to perform an "heavy" separation off the ground. The person who is "heavy" is not going to be an impressive exercise record. Muscle development is not evident and it will be over before the age of forty with the herniated disc!! !

Let's delve into the pectoral issue that was previously mentioned.

As we've observed the altered arrangement of the vertebral column as well as the clavicles causes the shortening of the pectoralis great that is enclosed within itself and is in a position of not extending or contracting throughout the full range of motion, losing as much as 50 percent in strength.

If we place the bar with a heavy workout on the bench, and then grips at the bar using a the grip supine, we aggrave the posture that is incorrect and the result will be shrinking the pectoralis great that will take on with the smaller pectoral a round shape. Furthermore, hypertrophy, or, more specifically shorter pectoralis major and of the latissimus dorsi muscle will increase the tendency to internalize and lower shoulders.

The best strategy to tackle this issue is:

Maintain all anterior and pectoral of the deltoid exercise to just a minimal and get rid of the parallels.

Eliminate tractions on the bar using a an supine grip, replacing them (if you're capable) by traction using an open grip, either forward or back, or sternal. Otherwise, you can use the machine for lats.

Incorporate a challenging and varied program for back pain which includes as exercises multiarticular base exercises: detachments (if there isn't any scoliosis) shakes, oarsman using a barbell, pulled onto the pulley, using a large grip bars and lying down.

Particularly, pulley pulls or rowers are best performed using an amount of weight that is less than the one typically employed. The attention of the muscles should be devoted to the stretching of the scapulae not the lifting of your arms to lift a huge weight.

We will now examine a frequent issue that is linked to posture the biceps during the classic barbell exercise. If shoulders are sagging forward and are weak, they already have weak. If we add weight, they'll be ripped forward and reduce the arc of the bar during the curl, and causing that the centre of gravity drop within the bust, instead of out. The overall form of the biceps is more prominent in the upper portion of your deltoid. If this is the case you may also be feeling at the end of a set of bicep curls using an exercise barbell, a trapezoid fatigue that exceeds the biceps as, in reality you're almost performing shakes. The solution is to adopt simple methods that put the biceps on a longer length and isolated. For instance, do the curl using dumbbells placed on a 45 degree inclined bench or the curl using barbells with your shoulders resting against the wall. Another typical occurrence of bad posture is the instability of the basin. This can cause negative consequences for all exercises, however specifically with the squat.

When it comes to issues with the squat's execution You never get bored and a perfect performance of the squat which includes lowering the pelvis to a point that the back isn't turned, will not leave the body free of injury. Actually, everybody takes note of the fact that the back of the lower part should not be round however nobody is aware of the fact that the back shouldn't even be arched !! A person who has an kyphotic stance and subsequent an adaptive lordotic lordosis that is secondary or secondary when performing the squat "naturally," raises the lower back and appears to be an ideal squat squat ace.

In actuality the case, excessive buckling, in addition to creating pressures that can be dangerous to the discs of the vertebrae, can cause pelvis's dislocation. What should we do, when a person suffers from scoliosis? The buckle that is required to complete"safe squat "safe squat" is going to come priced high the vertebral column that is in tension and anchored to the ground, will turn around itself in order to find its equilibrium and recreate the curves of its physiological function, by doing this, we sign up to the pension plans "safe hernia" and "cartilages consumed"!

In this instance an approach to this issue could be:

Alternate the squat exercise with the leg press or by extending your leg.

In the most grave cases, avoid all exercises where you are concerned that the force of your barbell puts a strain for the spine.

Make sure you select the right exercises that are suitable for your physical capabilities. This will allow you to go further in the direction of the development of your muscles than you obtain if you do exercises that are considered essential to build muscle, but risky for you to avoid at all cost.

The issues with posture that have been highlighted in the past have created an interest in a feature which is often neglected and the methods used to utilize a bodybuilding method which can be beneficial to those who don't suffer from serious issues and have an adequate level of general strength.

Chapter 11: Sprinting Vs. Jogging

In the quest to lose weight or becoming more fit, the majority of people are having a difficult time deciding whether to go for sprinting or jogging. Understanding the differences between the two is essential to make a decision. The speed of sprinting is fast and challenging on the body. However, running is more easy to master, particularly for those who are new to the sport because doing too much quickly can lead to injuries. It is important to know some things prior to making a decision on the best path or how to approach your workout. It is important to be aware of your preferences prior to your visit in order to make the right choice for you.

If you're trying to shed weight, then you're aware that reducing the amount of calories that you consume or burn is vital to the results you can expect and the amount of time you'll spend. Therefore, if you decide to do a workout, you must ensure that you burn off the maximum amount of calories during just one workout. Sprinting is the ideal option for those who you want to shed significant weight in a short amount of time. This is because sprinting boosts an increase in the amount of hormone growth (HGH) and helps in the growth of muscles that are lean. Therefore, sprinting causes an increase in metabolism that leads to the burning of stored fat. The result is the weight loss since the faster metabolism is likely to remain for a long time, regardless of any more exercise or a change in your exercise routine. Jogging aids in burning calories, but the quantities that are burned are considerably less and therefore it should be utilized to maintain your physique rather than for weight loss. Jogging is believed to be more beneficial as an everyday workout that helps keep the body fit or as a break between sprinting, allowing people to breathe.

Another factor to take into consideration when you are trying to lose weight is it is crucial to make sure that while you exercise, you're not losing muscle mass , but rather extra fat that is accumulating in your body. Running can use up muscles more to help you lose weight. Because it's usually performed for a long duration, it burns off calories that you have absorption and may cause a lower the body's mass index (BMI) because it strips the body of lean muscle and also leads to less bone mass. To be healthier running, it should be supplemented with other exercises like yoga and weight training to help combat difficulties caused by losing muscles. In contrast it is thought that sprinting can be the best way to lose extra body fat. While it is a lot of work on your body, it doesn't increase the muscle mass or diminish bone density. It improves lean muscles and bone density which contributes an increase to BMI.

In the present, everybody is very busy and seldom is there enough time for anything, or to squeeze in a whole exercise session. Thus, everyone is looking for a method of exercise which takes less time, however is still efficient. Because sprinting requires fast movements and is time-consuming, it can be done in a shorter amount of time. For instance, 100 meters can be accomplished in 20 minutes. Because sprinting is exhausting it is best completed by running for 50m at the maximum speed before walking or jogging to let your body relax before eventually sprinting the rest part of the way. A complete workout could comprise of about 8 sprints. While jogging, it is performed at a slow speed , which takes more time to achieve the same result as sprinting. The 45 mins of jogging equivalent to 10 minutes sprinting, in terms of the amount of calories burned.

Another crucial aspect to take into consideration when you are considering an exercise routine is the outcomes you'd like to achieve. This is the type of body you'd like to achieve from the exercise. This is also true for running and sprinting. Jogging, as mentioned previously, decreases the muscle mass of your body consequently, joggers have a body that isn't muscular or tight. It is often called'skinny fat' since a runners tend to be slim but carry larger body fat. This is why the jogger should supplement his/her running with other exercises which strengthen the muscles like weight lifting. Running, on the other hand, just burns off fats and the body becomes more muscular and athletic. This isn't an ideal thing for women who prefer an elongated, soft body instead of one that is strong and athletic. The bodies of sprinters have lower body fat and greater bone density. They also have larger muscles, and therefore weigh more than other people.

The best workout for running is one that combines both jogging and sprinting. This will allow you to last longer and not get tired too fast and burn more calories, which is the goal. Running for a long time is very stressful for the body, and jogging can allow one to relax to a certain degree. It is recommended to do this by sprinting one at a time for a certain distance, then when they are tired, they can start slow jogging and relaxing, before running another time for the remainder of the distance. Also, you can add an uphill run to increase the amount of calories burned, but it should only be done at least once a week since it is intense and could cause injuries.

Chapter 12: Poses To Stimulate

"The most essential items of equipment you require to practice yoga is your body and mind."

Rodney Yee

We've previously discussed the downward-facing dog, and it is among the most effective poses to incorporate into your arsenal if you're looking for energy, however there are other poses that are equally effective in gaining more energy. This chapter is dedicated to these poses, and if you're feeling a bit struggling to get your energy back, these are the ideal postures to help you get back your energy levels and feel more alive.

Mountain Pose and Floor Exercises

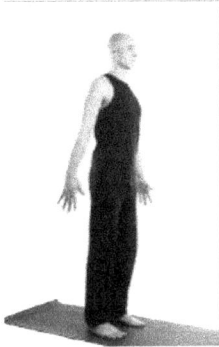

Place your mat on the floor with your feet on the floor. They should be level. Put your hands at your sides. The intention behind this posture is to strengthen your neck and shoulders. Your shoulders should be rolled forward and then come to a stop. Breathe. Reverse your shoulders, and then come to a stop. It is also a good posture to pay attention to your neck's position and how to how to keep your chin in and maintain your posture. It is possible to ask how this pose can be energizing, but it's the breath and the awareness in the pose that can do it.

From here, move to from there, you can move into the Extended Mountain posture. This is when you lift your hands over your head and then lean back as much as you are able to. Maintain this position, conscious that your stomach and tail end must be kept into. This method of tucking yourself into that assists in aligning your body so that energy flow smoothly through it. Relax deeply while you move your body.

From this point, you can bring your arms to the floor ahead of you while keeping your hands as close to the ground as they can in the waist region. To make this posture effective, you should have your hands facing toward the forward direction. If you are required bent your knees first to attain this, it's fine. Keep in mind that yoga isn't about pushing yourself beyond your limits but rather, learning your limits. This pose is called the Standing Forward Bend. It is excellent to improve circulation, stretch the tendons, and to feel an overall balance in your body. Once you're comfortable with this posture it is an important element of revitalizing your body.

There's a way to position yourself that can help you gain control of your breathing, and to do this, you'll need to lay face down upon the mat. Adjust your arms to ensure that your hands are close to your shoulders and your hands resting flat on the mat, facing towards the forward. To perform the modified long staff ensure that prior to the next exercise, you exhale deep. Standing on your knees, raise the front of your body while keeping your arms straight while your neck straight. Keep this posture, breathe in and let your body relax. Repeat this a few times. This will help strengthen stomach muscles and can give you energy, especially when you do it in conjunction with the workout that is below. It is the downward dog pose.

In the same posture as you did in the previous exercise breathe in and then move your head upwards, then straighten your arms and keep the extended chest position for a few seconds. Breathe and relax. This is a routine is required to repeat multiple times in order to reap the most benefits.

When you finish the routine, you'll be feeling energetic and may become a regular bedtime routine for those who want to feel more energy at night. Keep your yoga mat in the room to do these poses prior to the time you go to bed can really boost your sexual life. In addition you can also use them in conjunction with a midday meal to help you get your energy up for the afternoon or at mid-afternoon for help to get through the remainder days.

Practice, practice, and practice. While doing this you will notice that your body is more able to hold these poses with less effort. You'll become more flexible, and this is always sexy. Additionally, it makes you look younger and more energetic and keeps your waistline and your tail end in control. This is what yoga that is powerful is all about at its beginning. You'll discover that you have your own favorite poses that produce the results you want and that you incorporate them into your daily yoga practice. But, don't forget the benefits of meditation. A few minutes of mindfulness can really boost your energy levels and is a great thing to do in case you're feeling a little sluggish slightly mentally. It makes you feel energized and ready for everything.

Chapter 13: Lying Yoga Poses

Yoga poses that lie down are a fantastic way to stretch all parts in your body. They also help enhance digestion, and promote calmness. Here are a few yoga poses that can be done lying down:

The Fish Pose

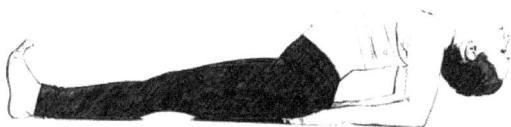

Benefits

• Reduces tension in your shoulder, neck, and throat.

* Reduces stress and irritation.

* Improves your posture

* It strengthens your upper back and your neck's back.

* Treatment of asthma and bronchial tubes and spasms

* Stimulates organs of your belly and throat.

Instructions

Begin by lying side on your floor (you may also lay on upon a yoga mat) and keep your knees bent while the feet resting either on the mat, or the floor.

Inhale and lift the pelvis slightly away from the ground (floor or mat) while slipping your hands and palms below the buttocks.

Inhale and hold the elbows and your forearms in a firm position against the floor or mat and then push the scapulas to the back. As you exhale, lift your upper torso and head off the mat/floor.

Then, you can continue to straighten your legs on the mat or maintain the knees bent. If you want to keep your legs straight, make sure that you keep your thighs very active. Then, press out with your heels. For 15-30 minutes, while breathing into your lungs slowly. When exhaling, be sure you lower the head and the torso toward the floor. Then, pull the legs up towards the belly, and then squeeze them a bit.

Corpse Pose (Shavasana)

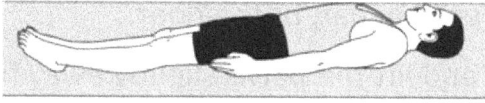

Benefits

* Takes you to the state of deep meditational repose

* Rejuvenates your entire body system

* Lowers levels of blood pressure and insomnia and anxiety

* Helps to keep your body in a steady state.

Instructions

Lay on your back, not the use of cushions or other props. If necessary, place the pillow in a small area below your neck and make sure that you shut your eyes.

Maintain your knees at a relaxed distance, while you completely relax your feet and knees.

Keep your hands in close proximity but a little away of your own body. Keep your hands open and open them to the sky. Relax your whole body by focusing on every part one after the one.

Begin by bringing your full attention toward your foot on the right side. Then, proceed to your right knee as well as all the other parts of the leg prior to turning your focus to the left leg. Continue to do this with other areas in your body till you are up to your head and have been able to relax all your body's muscles.

Keep taking slow, soft breaths. Allow your breaths to help become more relaxed. The breath you take in will help to you to energize your entire body, while the exhale helps to ease into relaxation. Remove your mind from any worries and concentrate solely on your breath and body. Be aware that you will not go to sleep.

After you've held this posture for 10 to 20 minutes and you can feel all parts of your body relaxing, slowly roll towards your right side while closing your eyes. Maintain that position for a few minutes or longer.

With the help by your left hand gently pull yourself into a seated position and take a few deep breaths, gradually become conscious of your surroundings and then gently let your eyes open.

Merry Baby Pose

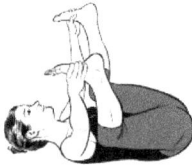

Benefits

* Extends your groins in the inner part of your body.

* Strengthens your back spine

* Calms your brain

* Aids in beating fatigue and stress.

* Increases the strength of your legs and widens your hips.

Instructions

Start by lying on your back and inhale while bringing both knees towards the chest. Then, pull the arms towards the insides of the knees. Hold onto the outside edges of both feet with both hands.

After that, tuck your chin in your highest position while making sure your head is to the ground. Then press the tailbone, as well as the sacrum into the floor while pushing the heels upwards and pushing your arms inwards.

Put your shoulders and lower back of your neck to the floor. Then, try to keep your back and your spine flat towards the ground. If you're in need of a greater flexibility in the hips, widen your legs slightly.

Deep breaths in and then fold your arms for around 4-8 breaths

To let go, exhale and let your legs and arms fall back down to the floor.

Pose for Wind Release (Pawanmuktasana)

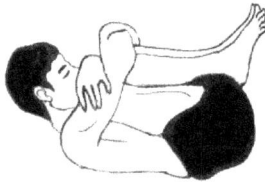

Benefits

* Improves digestion

* Massage your the pelvic region.

* Reduces menstrual problems and discomfort

Instructions

Lay on your back with your feet joined and your arms resting on your back.

Take a deep breath and, as you exhale then bring your right knee toward your chest.

Inhale deeply and, as you breathe out, ensure that you elevate your head as well as your chest off of the floor. Then, you can move your body to connect the chin to your right knee. Keep it for a few breaths.

Make sure to hold your knees while exhaling and let go of your grip when you take a deep breath.

Repeat the process with your left leg, then repeat using both legs.

Lying down on Sides (Vishnuasana)

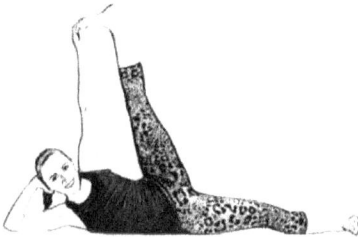

Benefits

The main reason to do this yoga posture is the fact that it stretch your pelvic joints.

* It also helps to tone your hamstrings.

Instructions

* Roll over and lay on your left side. Place your head on your right hand with your elbow resting on the floor.

* Lift your left leg and lower your left leg slowly down (Do this three times).

Make circles as you rotate the entire leg towards your pelvic joint.

* Repeat the exercise 5 to 6 times each in one direction, and in the opposite direction.

* Slowly lower your leg and then relax.

* Roll to lay down on your left and repeat the process then lie down on your back and unwind.

Body Twist Lieing Down (Jathara Parivartanasana)

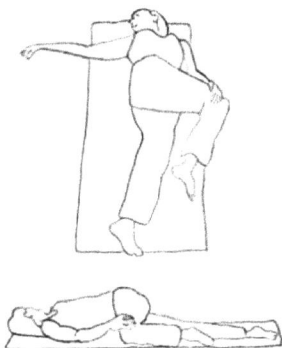

Benefits

* This will strengthen your back muscles.

* Provides deep relaxation to your body and mind.

* Stretch your quadriceps and spine.

Instructions

Relax on your back and spread out your arms from horizontal to your shoulders.

Relax your knees and pull your feet towards your hips. Keep your soles of feet on the floor.

Move your knees to the left till your left leg is on the ground. The right knee should rest upon your knees and the thigh.

Take the pose while feeling the stretch in your stomach, arms as well as your neck, back the groins and thighs.

Each time you exhale, ease your body deeper into the pose.

After a few minutes after a while, slowly rotate your head back towards the center, and then straighten your legs as well as your torso.

The Bridge Pose (Setubandhasana)

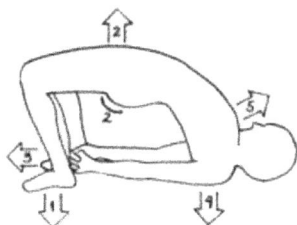

Benefits

* It strengthens your back muscles

* Instantly relieves your backache

* Lowers anxiety, soothes your mind and helps open your airways

Instructions

Lay on your back and relax.

Keep your ankles and knees to a straight position. lower your knees and keep your feet at a two-to-one distance from the floor. Set your arms on your body, with your palms facing up.

Slowly inhale and lift your upper and lower backs, lower backs and middle back off the floor. Keep your thighs in line with each others on the floor. make use of your shoulders to support your weight.

Interlace your fingers , then push your hands onto the floor to elevate your torso or utilize your hands to help support your back. Do this for two minutes and then exhale when you are ready to release the posture.

Plow Pose (Halasana)

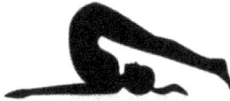

Benefits

* Tones your legs

* Enhances appetite and digestion

Keeps your spine flexible

* Increases the immunity

* Relieves symptoms of menopausal

Instructions

Start with the shoulder pose, and then exhale while you bend your hip joints, lowering the toes to the floor. You can also do this above your head. Keep your legs straight and your torso parallel to the floor.

While your feet are on the floor, pull your thighs up and the tailbone to the ceiling. Pull your inner groins in your pelvis. Keep drawing your sternum away from your chin and allow your throat to relax.

It is possible to release your hands from your back and spread your arms behind you on the ground, against your legs. Hold your hands in a tight circle and push your arms towards your back as you try to push your thighs upwards towards the ceiling.

To leave, put your hands behind then return to your starting position, and then as you exhale, you can roll towards your back, or let yourself go when you exhale.

18. Shoulder Stand (Sarvangasana)

Benefits

* Boosts blood flow to the central nervous system as well as the brain.

* Balances metabolism

* Aids in easing mild depression.

* Tone shoulder and arm muscles.

Instructions

Lay on your back, and keep your hands at your side. By making a single motion you can lift your back, buttocks and legs until you are to a high position on your shoulders. Utilize your hands to help support your back. The elbows should be moved towards one the other, and be sure to move your hands along the back, inclining toward the shoulder blades.

Keep your legs in a straight line and raise your legs toward the ceiling. Bring your big toes straight over your nose. Then, put your toes on the floor and be aware of your neck. Do not press your neck against the floor. Maintain your neck's strength by gentle tightening your neck muscles. Bring your sternum toward your chin. Continue to take deep breaths and hold them for 30-60 seconds.

Chapter 14: Effects Of Sitting

I

It has been stated it is said that "sugar is to teeth what sitting does for the spinal."

It's true. Sad yet real.

One of the most important reasons we sit is that our muscles that support our posture throughout our back start to relax.

If that occurs, that weight on our body is transferred directly into the spine's structure.

In the middle of the vertebrae that make up our spine, there are disks that function as shock absorbers.

With all the stress of the upper part of our body onto our spines and disks, with time our disks begin to dry out and then degenerate.

Every now and then we meet patients at my chiropractic clinic who have never had prior signs or symptoms, but suddenly, they must come in due to their lower back is "locked into." Their discomfort did not occur following a strenuous sport or painting their entire home or after doing an easy task like taking a piece of paper that fell on the floor.

The X-ray shows degeneration in the joints and disks that connect their vertebrae. The degeneration has occurred with time and without any pain.

The reality is that we weren't made to sit and stare at computers all day. We were made to move and we have to!

When we work for a long time such as at a computer for instance our shoulders can move upwards. In time, this can shorten the pec muscles. The pec muscles connect our breastbone, sternum, or to our shoulders.

As the muscles get shorter, our shoulders begin to move inwards.

Another thing that happens, particularly when we are sitting for a large portion of the day it is that we begin to adopt what's known as forward head position.

It's a pity that I see this happening more and more for children, even before they reach at the age of 10! It is a lot to do with the time they spend with electronics.

The time we spend using our mobiles.

The time you spend texting.

The time you spend playing video games.

Children are seated all day at school, and then coming back to their homes to complete their homework, play video games , and utilize their devices.

By putting your head in a forward position, the face shifts to the side and the head's weight starts to pull downwards on your spine.

If we have a forward-facing head posture If our head moves in a single inch forward it increases the weight of our head up to 10 pounds over our neck and our upper back!

Two inches of forward head posture for 12 pounds of head weight is equivalent 32 pounds of tension on your neck and the upper back.

Do you think that this could be the reason for some of your neck discomfort?

Imagine if I handed you a bowling ball , and I said that you were required to keep the bowling ball in your hands for two minutes. Would it be more comfortable to keep that bowling ball straight over your head? Or would it be more comfortable to place it before you with your arms extended?

It would be quickly if you had to keep it away from your body because the lower and mid back muscles as well as your arms would tire.

It's exactly what is happening to your muscles in your neck as well as your upper back.

It's not very easy to put the bowling ball above your head. However, what allows our body to keep our head straight is the fact that it was designed to do so.

Our necks have naturally curving lines to it. From an engineering point of view it's stunning to look at it as a structure that supports weight our neck curves, or curves under the surface of our skull to hold the weight of our head.

If we are sitting for too long and allow a forward posture of our head to develop over time it will result in the reverse of our natural curve in the neck.

Poor.

If we start to lose the natural support arc that holds the weight within our necks, it will usually cause muscular tension around your cervical back, the upper back, and at the base of your the skull. It can also cause tension headaches or discomfort in the shoulders.

Really, think about it for a second you feel that the ball's weight is moving upwards. The only thing you can do keep your chin from sliding down towards your chest is those neck lower back, upper back and upper shoulder muscles that are contracting and working harder to stay straight.

Because this condition is a gradual process over time, you become accustomed to muscles that are tight. You aren't aware at first that your movement range isn't quite as. Then you'll be able to turn your head left or right, or look upwards or downwards or turn your head towards your shoulders.

The other thing you may not feel initially, is the loss of curvature in your neck is placing pressure on the spinal cord. This could negatively impact the information that is transmitted between your body and brain.

Head posture that is forward and that head's weight being distributed to the front, can negatively impact your respiration (the quantity of exhalation and breathing you take from your lung.

Your breathing will become slow and shallow.

The capacity of the lungs can be reduced substantially.

Here is a complete list of other signs that may develop due to the forward position of the head:

* Chronic chronic (neck, shoulder lower back, upper and middle back, lower back)

* Jaw (TMJ) tension and dysfunction together with the teeth clenching

* Over time, arthritis develops in the joints and vertebrae of the neck.

* Nerve irritation due to inflammation, as well as the potential for disc impingement and degeneration of the neck vertebrae. This can cause sensations of numbness or tingling within the hands or arms.

* Reduced range of motion

* Migraines and tension headaches

* Reduced overall height

* Muscle spasms and tight and sore neck and chest muscles.

* Mouth breathing/ Sleep apnea

* Inadequate regulation of blood pressure

Chapter 15: The Risks Of Sitting

It's so widespread that we don't think about the extent to which we're doing it. Because all of us are doing it, it does not be a thought to us that sitting is unacceptable. The talk by Nilofer Merchant at TED 2013.

100 years ago when we were grazing in fields or working in factories, heart disease were largely unheard of. Since we're not able to freely roam the fields until the end of time and we have to take a stand for the right of standing. The act of sitting is not the primary reason behind all of these health risks and is instead the main cause for physical inactivity, which is the cause of numerous health issues that we are facing in the present.

Here are the actual risks of sitting for hours on end.

Weight gain and obesity

If you spend an extended period of time sitting during the day might notice that weight gain becomes an issue. When the body slows down when it is in a sitting posture, it is slowed down. Calories burn at a lesser rate when the majority of the muscles aren't engaged.

It is possible to snack at our desks throughout the day. This can mean empty calories are consumed, but not burning off. Many people have lunch at their desks! Making time for healthy snacks and meals may not be an ideal choice and your body weight and general health may suffer as a consequence. It is evident that people who have an active, sedentary life style are more likely be suffering from weight gain.

Accelerated Aging

The research published in The British Journal of Sports Medicine suggests that prolonged periods of sitting reduces your length of your Telomeres. They are DNA-caps at the ends of our chromosomes. every time a cell divides within our bodies and telomeres shrink, they become smaller and less. As we age, the natural process can lead to the telomeres becoming so short that cells are unable to more divide. Certain diseases or habits may change the size of our telomeres, too and accelerate the development, elevating the likelihood to be affected age-related ailments. One of these behaviors can be attributed to sitting.

MUSCLE DEGENERATION

Mushy Abs

While you stand or move , or even sit upright the abdominal muscles help keep your body upright. When you sit in the chair, they are inactive. The tightening of back muscles and the abdominal muscles that are tight create the "axis-of-evil" that affects the mid-section of the body. This can cause damage to the natural arch of the spine, frequently leading to back discomfort.

Tight Hips

Flexible hips aid in keeping you in a good posture, however those who are prone to stumbling rarely stretch the hip flexors muscles in the front, which causes them to become too tight and short, which limits movement along with stride length.

Limp Glutes

Take a seat and try to your butt (you most likely like doing this if there's nobody around but I'm not going to be judging if you don't). Do you feel as if it's an unflattened water balloon? The glutes of our bodies aren't designed to feel this way. The act of sitting requires your glutes to perform absolutely nothing and they are conditioned to it. The weak glutes can affect the stability of your body, your ability to move off and your ability to keep the normal pace of walking.

LEG DISORDERS

Poor Circulation in Legs

Long durations of time causes a decrease in blood circulation, which causes fluids to build up within the legs. Ailments can be swollen and varicose veins all the way to blood clots.

Soft Bones

Activities like walking and running cause leg and hip bones to get stronger and more dense. Researchers have linked the recent rise in cases of osteoporosis due to the absence of physical activity.

FOGGY BRAIN

Moving muscles move fresh oxygen and blood to the brain, and trigger the release of a variety of mood-enhancing and brain-boosting hormones. If we sit for long periods of time it slows everything down.

STRAINED the NECK

If the majority of your time is at your workplace desk continuously moving your neck towards the keyboard or bending your head so that you can hold your phone when you type could stress the neck vertebrae and lead to constant imbalances, and possibly vertigo.

BACK

The neck isn't the only one to slouch. The forward motion of slumbering can strain back muscles and shoulders too, especially the trapezius muscle, which joins the shoulders and neck.

BAD BACK

Flexible Spine

As we move around, the soft discs between vertebrae stretch and contract like sponges absorption of new blood as well as nutrients. When you sit for an extended period, discs get squashed differently. Collagen forms a hardened layer around ligaments and tendons which could result in a variety of back issues.

Disk damage

Sitting for longer periods of time puts you at a higher risk of developing herniated disks.

HEMORROIDS

Yup. We all not be happy however, if you do get them, it's a serious issue. Hemorrhoids are caused when the veins that surround the anus become inflamed that can lead to bleeding, itching, and itching. Who are most vulnerable to this issue? Truckers. And what do they do the majority often? You've guessed it ... the are seated for long durations.

A LOT OF SLEEPING HAS been linked to a variety of illnesses.

Sitting too long can lead to hypertension and blood pressure, as well as high blood sugar levels.

Sitting too long can lead to a bad mood

If you are seated for too long in your job, then you may not be as content as you might be. Individuals who sit for prolonged periods of time tend to experience depression or anxiety as per the Association for Psychological Science. The people who sat under three hours per day experienced fewer symptoms.

Going to the gym does NOT END THE NEGATIVE effects of sitting

The most troubling thing is the fact that spending a few minutes each week in the gym or engaging in vigorous or moderate activity isn't enough to reduce the risk.

People who spend for more than 3 hours each day on TV or browsing through the Internet are 64 percent more likely of heart-related disease. For those who are sitting for more than three hours and exercise, they are about the same weight as those who do not. If you train for 30 minutes, and then you spend most of the time not exercising it's like taking a multivitamin, and then taking a meal of French fries and Ice cream for the remainder of the day.

It's not just the Office

For many of us, averaging 8 hours per day at our jobs is a necessity. However, it's those extra hours working from home which can be the cause of our demise. One study examined people who sat less than 2 hours per day watching television or other screen-based entertainment to those who spent more than four hours per day on screens for recreational purposes. People who spent more time on screens included:

* A 50% greater risk of dying from any reason

* More than 125% more likely of incidents that are associated with heart disease, like the heart attack or chest pain.

Chapter 16: Perform The Yoga Poses Listed Below.

Warm-Up Exercises

Warm-up exercises are essential because they aid your mind in seamlessly transition into yoga routine. If you are a beginner you might need to do warm-up postures throughout your yoga class so don't avoid doing them throughout the entire week.

Warm-up yoga exercises strengthen your shoulders and the groin and lower back, as well as the back, and hips. This is a full-body yoga warm-up that you could do as a stand-alone exercise or in conjunction with other warm-up routines discussed in the following section.

While performing this workout, make sure that you use soft "fluid movements" which are a perfect combination of slow, deep breathing. To achieve more powerful and lasting outcomes, you should hold each stretch for around 1 or 2 breaths. If you are suffering from neck, arms, or back injuries, be cautious as failing to stretch could cause further damage.

1. The most effective way to do this is to start in the simple posture. In this pose, keep your shoulders low and to your back, your spine lengthened, and the chest is open.

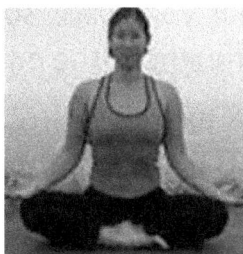

2. Take a deep breath , then gently lift your fingers to the ceiling. With your shoulders lowered and back, bring your hips down and touch the fingertips.

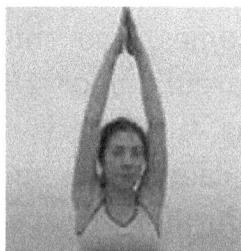

3. Inhale and then turn your body forward with your palms in the ground. Turn your spine around and relax the head and elbows.

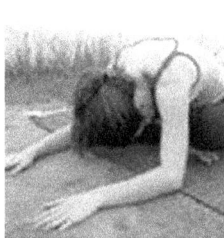

4. Inhale and then lift your fingers to the ceiling. Keep your shoulders down and to the back, with your hips are firmly anchored on the ground.

5. Begin to exhale while you turn to the

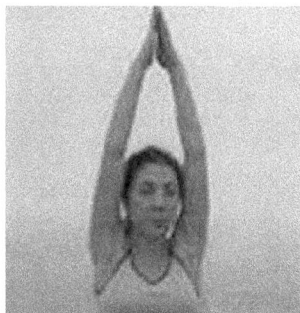

left. Place your left hand on your right knee, and place your right hand behind your back. Check the right shoulder and to the side behind your back. Maintain your spine's length and your shoulders back.

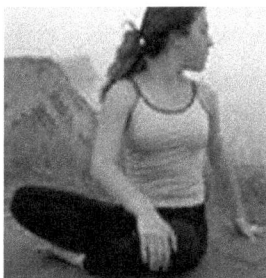

6. Breathe deeply and raise your hands toward the ceiling. Similar to before, keep your shoulders back and down. Additionally, make sure that your hips are firmly anchored towards the floor.

7. Inhale and then twist to the left. Place the right hand on the left knee, while placing put the hand of your left behind

your back. Check the left shoulder and then behind your back. Your spine must be straight and shoulders back.

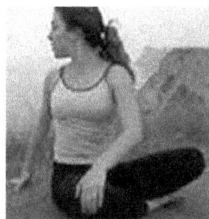

8. Inhale and raise your fingertips towards the ceiling. Keep the hips firmly planted to the floor, while bringing the shoulders to the side and back.

9. Exhale again and turn the left hand toward the floor. Then, move the hand toward the left. Reach out with the right fingers , and then lower the left arm as far as you are able to bear. Keep your chin away from the chest, and place the left arm should be placed over your right ears.

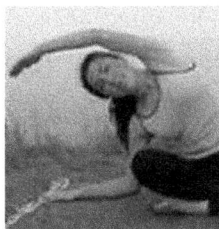

10. With your shoulders lowered and to the back Take a deep, gentle breath, and reach towards the ceiling with your fingers.

11. Breathe in, then turn your right hand toward the floor and then arch towards the left. Reach through your left hand and then bring your right elbow as close to the

floor as much as you can. Keep your chin off your chest. Keep your right arm above your left side.

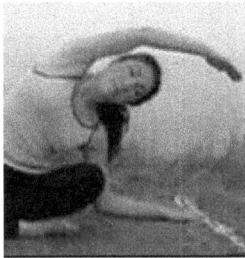

12. Take a deep breath, then gradually lift your fingertips toward the ceiling. When you exhale, bring your hands in the direction of forward movement and then turn your spine. Let your head drop when you extend your fingers out the fingers.

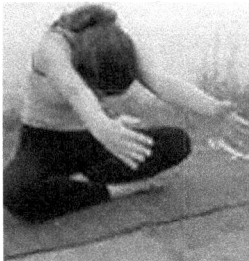

13. Breathe deeply and place your arms behind your. Make sure to extend your fingers to bring the shoulder blades in and then press them forward into your chest while looking towards the sky.

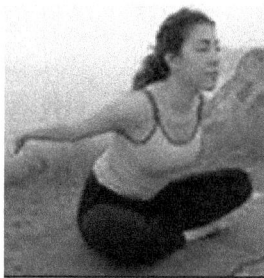

14. Breathe deeply and put your hands on your knees or on the ground. While bringing your shoulders back and back, gently pull your spine back to the neutral posture.

15. After that you are able to repeat the warm-up routine or, alternatively begin the asanas described below.

Standing Asanas

Asanas that are performed during standing yoga can helps align your body and feet because they relax your hips as well as strengthen your back. They stretch your legs and improve the range of motion. As well, standing yoga poses provide other benefits including assisting digestion, improving circulation of blood, and helping to lose weight. Alongside these physical advantages, a handful of the asanas that are performed during standing yoga are able to provide spiritual and mental advantages.

Let's look at a handful of these exercises and the advantages you will reap by doing these exercises:

1. Mountain Pose

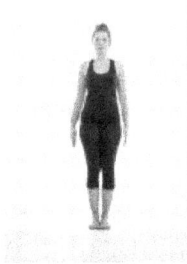

This posture is the basis of standing postures. By regularly practicing, you can improve the height of your body and improve your posture. In this posture the vertebral column of your spine and your heart are straightened, and the legs and arms are strengthened to combat fatigue. The pose also helps to improve stability and help focus to be in the present (mindfulness).

To learn the mountain pose to practice the mountain pose, follow these steps:

1. Place your feet on the floor and stand up straight. feet together to ensure that you are equally ground your feet.

2. Lift the head up and out by bending the top of your head.

3. Lift your thighs, and then continue to lengthen them by bending the four edges of the waist. While doing this, lengthen the spine , and breathe easily.

2. Triangle

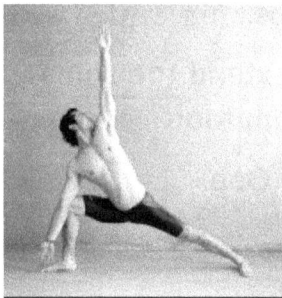

The triangle pose helps improve your balance, works your hamstrings and inner thighs and also allows your body to expand. If you practice enough you will be able to achieve the flexibility needed in this posture.

1. Keep your feet spread apart. Then, slightly twist your left toes , allowing your right thigh wide. Continue until you reach your right toes straight to the side.

2. Then you should ground your feet, and then pull your legs up, making sure your legs are straight.

3. Widely spread your arms to shoulder height. Then begin rolling your front of your thigh, and proceed to hinge the front of your hips.

4. Try to extend the spine in the direction of your front foot.

3. Warrior One

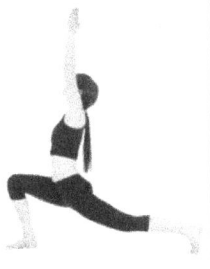

The warrior's pose relaxes and eases the mind of a stressed one it increases stamina and helps strengthen ankles and legs.

1. Begin with an upward-facing dog position and then move your right foot in front of the hands.

2. Inhale the left heel and, as you exhale raise your arms and the torso. Check that the foot on your left side is aligned to the rear of your back arch of your foot.

3. Keep the front of your knee directly over your ankle. Move both hips inwards, and then pull your tailbone downwards while pulling your ribs back.

4. Check that your hip's rear is facing forward, not to the side. Then, turn the back of your feet around 45 degrees.

5. Repeat the same pose on the opposite side.

4-Half-Moon Pose

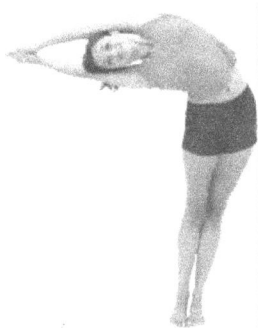

The practice of this pose can stretch the stomach's sides and strengthens the abdominal muscles and assists in burning belly fat. Half-moon poses also tone the inner and outer thighs , as and the buttocks for every gender. For a good practice the pose, adhere to these guidelines:

1. Begin by standing up and put your hands together. Place your hands on your head and bind the palms together. It is recommended to extend your stretch by reaching towards the ceiling.

2. Breathe deeply and slowly turn your hips sideways as you hold your hands in a tight position.

3. Keep your elbows straight and straight. Avoid bent forward until you feel the "stretch sensation" which comes from your fingers and thighs.

4. After a couple of minutes, breathe deeply and then return to the original standing position.

5. Repeat the half moon pose from the opposite side.

Chapter 17: The Theory Of Bodyweight Exercises!

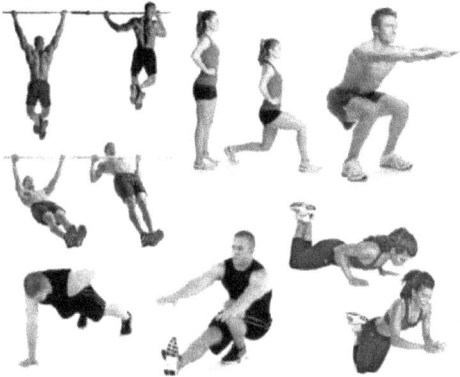

The exercises that are done with body weights are thought of as strength training, and this type exercise isn't required any additional weights or free ones. It is among the most commonly practiced fitness regimens by the majority of people around the world. The weight of the body provides resistance to their movements. This means that they utilize their own body weight to strengthen muscles and improve their power, strength and to build a more leaner body. The practice of strength training can be described as a kind of physical exercise that makes use of your body's energy to provide many advantages. It helps improve the physical condition, fitness and overall health. These exercises help in strengthening muscles, enhancing the cardiovascular system, improving the athletic ability, helps with weight loss and helps maintain overall fitness and health.

The most frequently practiced exercises using body weight include pushups sit ups, pull ups such as crunches, lunges, and many more. When these workouts are done regularly they can be extremely beneficial in increasing endurance, strength and general flexibility. This is definitely one of the best ways to build your body efficiently and increase strength, power , and pave way to a slimmer, healthier body.

The most common misconceptions is that extravagant or sophisticated equipment is required for a stronger and more leaner body. This is an untruth that has been completely dispelled. The bodyweight exercise is ideal for those looking to show off their physique without having to shell out huge sums. Integrating weights or body exercises into your daily workout routine is the best method to boost the development and growth that your physique.

Chapter 18: Food And Yoga

Food and diet are essential to yoga. The consequences of poor nutrition and unhealthy eating manifest their presence in a sloppy appearance, and in poor mental and physical behavior. Based on yoga's principles eating, food is classified as Rajasic, Tamasic and Sattvic that is an old-fashioned way to describe the Good as well as the Bad and Ugly.

* SATTVIC Yoga Foods

They are meals that are made fresh and prepared using only minimal spice or seasonings. They retain their nutritional value because they are prepared with minimal effort. One of the best tasting and nutritious foods that can provide significant benefits to general health of your body is Sprout. The yoga principles highly recommend eating Sattvic food.

* RAJASIC Yoga FOODS

These foods are frequently referred to as meals for kings or those with active or inactive temperaments. An array of different foods prepared in various ways -

baked, fried or spiced, make up this category of yoga foods. Additionally, this category includes alcohol, processed beverages and sweets. In general, these foods add weight and fats for the body. They cause feelings of unease following eating, which can lead to an energy level that is low.

* TAMASIC Yoga FOODS

This includes non-vegetarian as well as vegetarian dishes that include salts, hot seasonings and extra spices. According to general opinion they create a sense of slackness for those who eat them. The foods that fall into this category can result in a rough and intolerant temperament.

Yoga Diet - Foods to Avoid

1. Margarine, poor-quality oils, and animal fats

2. White sugar and white flour

3. Foods with a lot of spice

4. Foods that are old, stale, and over-heated food items

5. Genetically engineered food products

6. Foods that have been microwaved and irradiated

7. Fish, eggs, and even meat

8. Fried food items

9. Dairy products from the factory farm

10. Canned food items (excepts tomatoes that are canned naturally fruit, vegetables, and vegetables)

11. Processed, artificial foods

12. Artificial sweeteners

13. Tea, coffee as well as alcohol, tobacco and all stimulants

Yoga Diet - Foods to Eat

1. Natural sugars, such as maple syrup, molasses honey, and Jiggery

2. Whole grains, such as wheat, oats and rice

3. Pulses and lentils

4. Fresh juices, particularly the lemony type, as well as teas and water

5. Fenugreek basil, mint and turmeric. Coriander, cumin, cardamom, fennel as

well as ginger, cinnamon and other sweet spices

6. A little salted or roasted nut like sesame, pecans as well as coconuts, walnuts, and almonds

7. Dairy products include cottage cheese as well as yogurt, ghee, and milk from dairy animals that are well-treated

8. Cleared butter (ghee) as well as any other kind of natural plant-based oils like sesame, olive, and sunflower

9. Fruits that are sweet and sweet, fresh of all kinds are best eaten whole

10. All kinds of vegetables, but especially green leafy varieties.

Things to Take Note of:

The way you cook and consume your meals is as important as the food you consume. Eat and cook your meals in a loving and mindful manner like you perform yoga on the mat. Yoga practitioners who practice using yoga principles are aware of this type of thinking. Eating or chatting with your food when you're distracted anger or upset may result in negative effects such as stomach upset. Even if you're eating at a restaurant and the food that is served to you isn't your typical yoga-style diet eating the food, praising it and knowing that you want to eat the food and then eschew the rest of it can turn it into positive dining experience.

The key is moderation

As with every healthy eating plan, a yoga diet that emphasizes moderate and balanced eating is crucial. It is not just related to the quantity of food consumed but also to the spices and other flavors which are present in it. A lot of grease, strong spices , or an overdose of spices should not be included in a yoga regimen and should be limited to fresh, natural food items are the best for nutritional value. Infusing your taste buds with too much food or your food plate puts an enigma on your thoughts and mood.

When is the best time to eat?

Yoga experts strongly recommend that you avoid eating food for 2 up to 3 hours prior to an exercise class. Many yogis also recommend eating foods that are safe for your stomach and digestive system. Some suggestions include things like toasty whole wheat bread, hummus, rice, vegetables low-fat yogurt, apples oatmeal, and pears. Foods for pre-workout snacking should be with a low glycemic score and beware of sugars and simple carbs like white bread, donuts and sweets.

Rule Exclusions

Because of health concerns and food allergies along with other issues A strict diet of yoga won't be suitable to everyone. However, this is not a problem since there are variations in the yoga diet that allow yogis to eat fish or meat in order to remain focused and healthy. The most important thing is to pay attention to your body and adjust your diet to your body's demands instead of adhering to a strict diet plan that can cause you to feel sick tired, weak or fatigued.

Chapter 19: Body Butter And The Powers Of Body Butter

If you're suffering from back pain, you may just want a refreshing natural lotion that you can apply more often and, in the majority of cases, offering a pleasant smell. This is exactly the reason these natural body butter recipes can be used for. Apply them all over your back, and they're also beneficial to other muscles suffering from discomfort as well. They are designed to be applied as lotions, and has much less consistency than balms. They're however, generally thought of as less effective, and can't be used to treat acute back pain relief.

#1 Lavender Body Butter

Lavender body butter is easy to make and also has a pleasant smell. Lavender has properties that help decrease anxiety, panic and anxiety. Back pain that is chronically afflicted is usually caused by the tension in muscles caused by external factors that cause stress. The benefits of lavender body butter will allow you to get rid of the back pain naturally.

Ingredients:

1. 1/4 Cup Shea Butter

2. 1/2 Cup Mango Butter

3. Half Cup Coconut Oil

4. 1 Cup Lavender Flowers, Dried

Directions:

1. Utilizing blender, mix your lavender flowers with a high speed until they're more fine.

2. Pour the coconut oil into an enormous pot set over the flame at a low temperature, then pour your lavender flowers making sure that they're properly mixed in. Let it sit at a low temperature for 3.5 hours, then remove the flowers. Be aware that you need to stir it frequently to avoid it to catch fire.

3. Utilizing a double boiler, blend all the oils and butters. Be aware that you should

stir frequently on low heat if do not want your shea butter to get gummy.

4. Let it chill in the refrigerator for few hours before removing it and beat it. Place the butter in airtight containers. Apply it to the sore areas according to the need.

#2 Body Butter Whipped Magnesium, Chamomile

If you have sufficient magnesium, you'll be less likely to suffer from back pain that is constant Additionally, it may assist in easing any discomfort that may occur in flare-ups. Roman lavender flowers can assist in relieving soreness because of their anti-inflammatory capabilities. Once you've infused your oil the soft and gentle body cream has a fantastic aroma and is easy to apply. You can apply it on as you would any other cream however often you'd like on a daily basis.

Ingredients:

1. 1 Cup Shea Butter

2. 1 Cup Coconut Oil

3. 1/4 Cup Magnesium

4. 1 Cup Chamomile Flowers, Dried

Directions:

1. Pour the coconut oil in an enormous pot, and infuse the chamomile flowers by simmering at a low temperature for 2.5 hours, mixing it regularly.

2. Remove the flowers of chamomile, then mix all the ingredients in a double-boiler, and let it melt over a the flame at a low temperature while mixing until it is all combined.

3. Let it be cool down in the fridge for while before removing it and beat it until it looks like butter. Place the butter in airtight containers. Apply it to the sore areas whenever needed.

#3 Body Butter #3 Body Butter Peppermint and Lavender

It's well-known that lavender is a great remedy for back pain If you mix in peppermint leaves and cream for your body, it will make an extremely potent concoction. It'll provide a cool sensation which will reduce stiffness and swelling.

You will definitely be reducing tension as well. You can infuse coconut oil over a prolonged period of time for an even more potent result.

Ingredients:

1. 1/2 Cup Lavender Flowers, Fresh

2. 1/4 Cup Peppermint Leaves, Fresh

3. 1 Cup Coconut Oil

4. 1 Cup Shea Butter

Directions:

1. In a large pan let your peppermint and lavender to infuse into the coconut oil, heating it over at a simmer over 3.5 hours. Be sure to mix the mixture frequently to ensure there is no sticking, then strain the herbs and allow the oil that has been infused to remain.

2. Mix the oil infused with the shea butter in a double saucepan at a low heat until it melts and mixes.

3. Place it in an enormous bowl, then whip it once and then is then placed in the refrigerator to cool.

4. Once it is cool then take it out and whip it until it's soft and soft. Scoop it up into airtight containers to use.

#4 Body Butter #4 Body Butter Thyme and Ginger

If you're not averse to the smell of a cream for your body which isn't as pleasant This scent of Thyme and Ginger combination could be the right thing to rid yourself of that kink that has been lingering within your lower back. Although it may not be as powerful than some of the other butters for body however it has the essential properties needed to ease back pain.

Ingredients:

1. 12 Cup Thyme, Fresh

2. 4. Tablespoons Ginger Grated

3. 1 Cup Coconut Oil

4. 1/4 Cup Shea Butter

5. 1/2 Cup Cocoa Butter

Directions:

1. Incorporate your coconut oil into the pot of a large size, and mix the thyme and

ginger in it, simmering at a low temperatures for 4.5 hours while mixing it regularly.

2. Clean out all herbs, preserving the oil that was infused. With a double boiler mix the cocoa and shea butters and the oil that you have infused.

3. Let it chill in the refrigerator for while before you take it out and beat it. Place the butter in airtight containers. Apply it to the sore areas whenever needed.

#5 Body Butter #5 Body Butter Lavender and Sandalwood

Like many of the other blends we've discussed, any blend that contains lavender will impart a soothing scent to it. This body butter with a pleasant scent is yet another combination of stress relieving that you can make to ease the strain on your back. Essential oil of sandalwood is the main ingredient to eliminate anxiety and anxiety. Make this body cream and note the improvement you feel in your back after applying it.

Ingredients:

1. 1/2 Cup Lavender Flowers

2. 20 Drops Sandalwood Essential Oil

3. Half Cup Coconut Oil

4. 1 Cup Shea Butter

Directions:

1. Combine the coconut oil as well as lavender blooms into the pot in a large bowl and cook on a low flame for 3.5 hours while mixing frequently.

4. Clean out all herbs and keep the oil that was infused. Utilizing a double boiler, blend the cocoa and shea butters with the oil that has been infused.

2. Remove the heat and pour into the bowl of a medium size. Add the essential oil of sandalwood and mix thoroughly. Whip it before placing in the refrigerator to cool.

5. Let it cool in the fridge for two hours, then take the butter and beat it. Place the butter in prepared airtight containers. Apply it to the sore areas whenever needed.

Chapter 20: Gymnastics In The Airplane And For Office Employees

The commonality among passengers on planes and office workers is that both groups of people spend the majority of their time sitting and this is detrimental to the human body, especially joints and spine.

In order to keep your back in the proper straight position in order to support your lower lumbar bend (lordosis) from the seat of the passenger is incredibly difficult. Even a plaid-colored roller, which is offered to a passenger, and set under the lower back doesn't always help the back. Intervertebral discs and joints that are overloaded at the final stage of the flight or when you are completing baggage claim may cause retribution to the person who owns them with extreme pain, or the appearance of disc herniation.

In this scenario in such a situation, it is recommended to do the Heel isometric gymnastics workout (see the description below) is a great tool for the back. For those who are sitting it isn't an exercise but rather a position that must be held throughout the trip. The simple way to do this is to lift the heel off the floor as the sock stays in position.

If you're sitting right now and you are sitting down, try an experiment that is simple. Remove both heels from the floor, and allow your feet until they touch the floor, and then hold the position for at least a one minute. If until this point your back and your ribs were in a tense position at the time, then in the close to the end of this posture and with the heel ripped off the lumbar spine becomes straight and is easily maintained in the proper position. The reason is in the characteristics of the biomechanics in the human body. We will stick to the idea that having a straight back is simpler to hold a torn heel up and affixed to the weight.

In any case regardless, this "Heel" exercise lets you keep in the healthy, physiological position the most vulnerable area of the traveler's lower back. It is possible to pull off both heels at the same time or lift them one at a time one. You can lift and lower your heel and still secure it by putting it on the weight. In any event the isometric workout "Heel" won't cause your back pain at the end of your travel and avoid a trip to the pharmacy to purchase painkillers when you are in a foreign country.

If you've not eaten on the plane If you have not eaten, the workout "Press" is extremely beneficial (see the explanation below). Use two hands to press your abdominals and keep this tension for about 20-30 minutes. This workout strengthens the abdominal muscles wall, which stimulates digestion, and stops constipation from travelers.

When you travel on any plane in, sleep is always with the passengers and you need to find a suitable place and the right position for the head to rest in the passenger seat. Cervical vertebrae and discs that hold their heads in this awkward position are bound to are prone to suffering. So, isometric gymnastics for those traveling must include exercises to strengthen the neck. Isometric neck tension doesn't require much space and could be done even in the cramped seats of an aircraft.

To strengthen the neck spine it's sufficient to position the hands on the front of the head and then place them onto the forehead and and then on the sides of the head. Perform isometric tensions of the neck muscles by applying tension to arms. It's not necessary to show the exercises of your travel neighbor, however you'll be surprised when he decides to be able to join in your classes as well. An in-depth description of exercises is provided in the section on the cervical spine within the text.

Continue working on the neck. Following these exercises, shift your hands towards the lower area of the neck . Perform those exercise "Squeeze your neck muscles" as well as "Stretch your chest's fascia." These two exercises can help with the stagnation of lymphatic and venous flow within the neck and head tissues. and neck. All movements during these exercises are led downwards to the clavicles, which is the region where the lymph nodes are situated which collect fluid from the neck and head.

It is said that the neck has been "finished" The neck is "finished" and the attention of the traveler goes further down -- to the shoulder girdle, which is the shoulder blades and chest. Travelers, who are confined by the seat of a car or an aircraft, is offered two isometric gymnastics "Japanese greeting" and "Castle".

For this exercise you need to have your palms before you and you will try to squeeze them, then, separate two. The next part in these workouts is linked to stretching muscles. If you are sitting in a tight chair in the course of "Lock" to stretch the muscles in the back using the elbow is easy, then stretching the pectoral muscles during the workout "Japanese greeting" is quite challenging.

However, you could do at the very least some initial stretch of the pectoral muscles when you bend your elbows at the elbows and move them as far back as you can and bring the shoulder blades as close as is possible. The pectoral muscles being stretched in this manner is quite obvious. You can also repeat these exercises according to the specific description provided in the specific chapter of this book.

Which is the most comfortable seat to ride on? Sure, the more comfortable seat is the better choice. In many trains bus seats are tough and not covered with any kind of covering. We must develop anti-vandal design which are detrimental to passenger's comfort. Even in a comfortable seat in an airplane the four-hour flight can numb the pelvic region as well as the buttocks so that they literally become numb and lose their sensitivities. This is because the fat tissue of the buttocks can offer a benefit over the thinner ones: fat can soften and shield the muscles and nerves beneath including that sciatic nerve.

A slim person doesn't have this elastic and soft fat, and the weight of his body can easily be transferred to the nerves of the sciatic nerve. Nerve cell conductors along with their vessels get compressed and the patient is numb or weak on the side of the leg. This is not just painful, but also dangerous as the nerve is a highly sensitive organ and a disruption of blood circulation is very undesirable.

Another issue that can be aggravated by prolonged sitting causes irritation in the coccyx as well as its ligaments. It is the posture of sitting which causes stress to the ligament of sacrococcygeal. The stress of sitting can cause discomfort, particularly in the case of injury to the coccyx from having fallen on the buttocks in the past.

To avoid further stress of tail remnants from sitting for a long time, can be used for the exercise "Walking in buttocks". The essence of this move lies in the name:

while sitting in a chair at work or on an automobile, airplane and train chairs, you move the body from behind of the chair towards an edge on the side of the chair, and then back using the buttocks. To accomplish this, transfer your body weight to one buttock, then lift the otherand then shift around in the seat. Be sure to use your foot a little. When you've worked your buttocks, and put an amount of force to your hip joints and the lower lumbar region of your body, free the tailbone and you'll not be concerned about further periods of sedentary work.

Travelers can't be left out of hands. Even though we do not use our hands when we travel or move, practicing brush-hand exercises will help. This is because brushes contain a large amount of bioactive zones and points. The method of Chinese Acupressure and acupuncture, massage in accordance with the theories from the ancient Inca or Maya doctors - all utilize brushes as the most important instruments to improve the health.

It is necessary to know the positions of the points and zones as well as the treatment method as well as the entire philosophies of the technique. We won't go into complicated yin-yang relations, but make use of the brush in its entirety. Three exercises for tourists who is beneficial to do - "Fist fan", "Finger traction", "Squeezing fingers."

For the first time, squeeze your hands into a fist . Then make sure you hold your fist as tight as possible using a voltage of 10-30 seconds. After that, you can let your fingers open like fan, and then keep the tension for 10-30 minutes. Following that we stretch the joints, ligaments, and muscles. Learn how to do this with regard to travel.

Conclusion

Being active and exercising is one of the best ways to ensure bone strength. It's essential to take a walk or weight training and running every day to ensure your bones are healthy and free of any ailments. These exercises also help prevent loss of bone, which happens in time, but it can be controlled by a healthy diet and exercise.

Beware of a lifestyle that is sedentary particularly if you work at home. Be sure to discover ways to stay active as sitting for longer than 9 hours a day is likely to result in hip fractures as well as other issues. Utilizing the stairs instead of the elevator is a good beginning to ensure the proper maintenance of bone strength. Always make sure to strengthen your muscles harder to prevent the loss of bone.

The most important thing is to establish discipline in all your activities. Make sure you are focusing on improving your bones health and be sure you set goals for your longer-term strength of your bones. Consult your physician regularly and not just when you're experiencing problems in your joints or bones. Be aware that prevention is always better than treatment and bone ailments are not always easy to treat.

In this quick guide, you will discover the most important techniques to maintain the strength of your bones. There are many helpful suggestions you can find in particular to ensure your bones are healthy as you get older. In the end, your senior years will be the most difficult aspect of fitness.

The most enjoyable part is to discover delicious recipes to improve bone health. Perhaps, eating meals at home which contain calcium-rich foods is the most effective option in maintaining your teeth, bones muscles, nerves, and muscles in good shape. So, which suggestions in this book are intending to incorporate into your bone-health regimen?

www.ingramcontent.com/pod-product-compliance
Lightning Source LLC
Chambersburg PA
CBHW060331030426
42336CB00011B/1286